*To Kay,
with best wishes,
David*

HANNAH
Unmasked

Hannah Rose

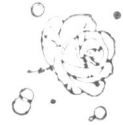

**written in collaboration
with David Mitchell**

Published by New Generation Publishing in 2022

Copyright © Hannah Rose 2022

First Edition

The author asserts the moral right under the Copyright, Designs and Patents Act 1988 to be identified as the author of this work.

All Rights reserved. No part of this publication may be reproduced, stored in a retrieval system or transmitted, in any form or by any means without the prior consent of the author, nor be otherwise circulated in any form of binding or cover other than that which it is published and without a similar condition being imposed on the subsequent purchaser.

ISBN   978-1-80369-306-4

www.newgeneration-publishing.com

New Generation Publishing

Dedicated to...

All who have helped me during a difficult period in lockdown

Acknowledgements

Susan Mitchell, yet again, for proof-reading

Howie Rose, for sorting my computer out at a crucial moment!

CONTENTS

INTRODUCTION 1
CHAPTER ONE: My New Home 3
CHAPTER TWO: Back in Florida 11
CHAPTER THREE: Another Turn for the Worse 16
CHAPTER FOUR: Rescue in the Car Park............................19
CHAPTER FIVE: 'Hannah Rose, News at Ten, Northwich Station' 24
CHAPTER SIX: A Wedding Guest in Tuscany 29
CHAPTER SEVEN: Stuck in the Mud 41
CHAPTER EIGHT: Tattoo or Not to Do? 44
CHAPTER NINE: Lockdown 47
CHAPTER TEN: Lockdown Routine 54
CHAPTER ELEVEN: Zoom! 62
CHAPTER TWELVE: A Welcome Break by the Sea 68
CHAPTER THIRTEEN: A Brilliant Family Christmas.........73
CHAPTER FOURTEEN: Managing My Team 78
CHAPTER FIFTEEN: Friends for Life..................................87
CHAPTER SIXTEEN: My Lovely Bunch of Roses 94
CHAPTER SEVENTEEN: Joanne..105
CHAPTER EIGHTEEN: The Joys of Online Shopping 109
CHAPTER NINETEEN: In and Around Politics.................114
CHAPTER TWENTY: Loving the Live Music 118
CHAPTER TWENTY-ONE: National Heroic Service........120

CHAPTER TWENTY-TWO: Three Chairs for Hannah!.... 127

CHAPTER TWENTY-THREE: The Joys and Perils of Keeping in Touch 130

CHAPTER TWENTY-FOUR: Thought-Provoking TV 135

CHAPTER TWENTY-FIVE: 'It was twenty years ago today…'.. 143

CHAPTER TWENTY-SIX: Milestones 151

CHAPTER TWENTY-SEVEN: Opportunities with Leonard Cheshire.. 155

CHAPTER TWENTY-EIGHT: Back to the Seaside 160

CHAPTER TWENTY-NINE: Meeting up – at last! 165

CONCLUSION 170

APPENDIX: Interview with the Leonard Cheshire Organisation, 2021... 171

'You have achieved more in your twenty years since you came out of hospital than many will in a lifetime.'

INTRODUCTION

I'm back with book number three and there's plenty of new stuff to tell you about! Both my previous books, 'Hannah Same Both Ways' and 'Hannah Moving On', have given me so much pleasure, particularly all the nice comments that people have said about them. Because of restrictions placed on us by the pandemic this third manuscript has been done over the telephone. One of the highlights of weeks and weeks when relatively little happened in my life has been my telephone chats with Sue and Dave Mitchell each Tuesday and Thursday afternoon. They were so therapeutic and became something to look forward to. I continued to drive Dave mad as I moved randomly from one subject to another! One moment we might be talking about iron infusion or training for carers when out of the blue would come,

'The red fish is alive! Oh, I'm so relieved.'
'Bye Barbara!'
'You should see Mabel. She's moulting like a trouper!'
or
'Doorbell, Claire! It must be another Amazon delivery.'

If there was a degree for waffling, I'd have a first! Many a time Dave will ask me to repeat what I've just said and I can't remember!

The COVID issue that has dominated our recent lives will feature heavily this time round. It has given me plenty of problems to deal with but, also, reasons to be cheerful. The book also looks back over the twenty years since I first went into Alder Hey Hospital in May 1999. The chapters are full of familiar faces as well as some new ones who have made a big impression on me.

CHAPTER ONE

My new home

'As it came to moving out of the home that I'd known all my life I just didn't know what to feel.'

At the end of 'Hannah Moving On' I was in the conservatory of my still relatively new home. Mum and Dad were with me as we took stock of where I had got to in my life and the significance of leaving the family home behind after seventeen years. I had loads of doubts and anxieties during the planning stage. There had been some huge decisions to make such as where I could reasonably live relative to all my current support and family and what the layout of my ideal house would look like. It is difficult to believe that it is now four years since I moved in and I absolutely love being here. I didn't think that I'd ever have such a big drive all to myself!

Surprisingly, the first night at my new home wasn't as weird as I thought it might have been. I had expected to feel sadder than I did but I adjusted quickly, carried along by the excitement! It must have been stranger for Mum and Dad, having their house to themselves for the first time in absolutely ages. It has worked out well for them, though. They have been able to convert my room in the garage to design the big modern kitchen that Dad, in particular, has always craved and it is unimaginable to think that my bed was once in there. They have been able to lock the front door regularly at night knowing that no one would be turning up for shifts. They have got their house back again.

Once the move had been sorted there were many decisions to make around the organisation of my domestic life and how my lovely team of PAs would operate. Moving from a base within my family home to my new house would mean a significant change of emphasis.

With Mum and Dad no longer being in the house overnight we set-up an on-call system to support the night shift should there be an emergency. I might need help, or one of the PAs might be unwell. Having a back-up in such circumstances would be reassuring. We have used this system several times since. That's not a lot, thankfully, but I was glad to have something in place as an insurance.

I was able to allocate a designated room for the PAs to base themselves in. This was a significant improvement on what I had been able to offer at Mum and Dad's which had been a much smaller space tucked between the kitchen and my bedroom. In their new base they can watch television, play DVDs or just read quietly. There is a lot of reading in between the required checks of my records, temperature or night bag.

I have a cosy lounge where I can operate lights and television through assistive technology. From my seat I like to be able to see the fire, the TV, the fish tank and Mabel, who is still my loyal four-pawed lovely Labrador companion! I love watching them all. My friend Alexa can confuse people because turning the fire light on can also turn the fan on! I have always loved garden time in the sunshine and have space front and back to sit in. At the front I might end up chatting to neighbours going past. I remember one example towards the end of February 2021. It was the first time I'd been able to sit out after the winter. Yay! I was going to take Mabel for a walk but there was a nice sun trap near the front door. I had a bit of lunch there and did some work before taking Mabel at around four o'clock. On the way back in I saw Thelma and Tony, from next door but one. We chatted for ages and by the end I was freezing! It was just like the start of spring and I loved being outside with them. Everything feels so normal at times like that.

The back garden is more private and I can sit out in my chair without being disturbed. I've had a new shed put up. There was a hedgehog underneath the old one! Down to more advanced technology now available to me I was able to send a video of the hedgehog to family and friends. I'll be saying much more about exciting developments in assistive technology later in the book!

One important consideration in the new house was the emphasis that needed to be placed on the many domestic duties required in any typical household. Previously, Mum and Dad had kept the house going. PAs were sometimes reluctant to interfere and tread on their toes when it was their property. My washing, for instance, would be mixed up with theirs and Mum was best placed to sort it out.

Now I had to make my own arrangements to keep the home ticking over. I was totally independent and had to ensure that there were no grey areas. Between myself and my caring team we had to think of the running of the house and the many practicalities involved such as keeping everywhere clean, washing, emptying bins, sorting the fridge and freezer out and feeding Mabel. We thought of job lists that could be ticked off each day or each week. That has been really helpful. We had to make adjustments and everyone bought in quickly to the new arrangements. My new house is now other people's work space rather more than previously.

There has been a significant change of emphasis in my daily eating habits. Despite all the improvements in my life eating is still one thing that I cannot do by myself although I have recognised the importance of a good diet for my welfare. Dad and Mum don't feed me often now. I was saying to one of the PAs before bedtime, 'Just imagine what it used to be like when I was at Mum and Dad's house. Four years ago they were doing everything for me. They would invariably provide my meals and often feed me. I ate what they ate. It's hard to imagine that now although Dad goes to LIDL on a Saturday night and gets me items which I add to his list, despite me having a supermarket delivery each week. I did have a go at him for no reason once when I asked him to get me some tuna. He came back with one tin. Now, I'm sorry but who buys just one tin of tuna? You'd buy a set. Jess and Naomi were laughing as I cried,

'One tin, one tin of tuna? Who buys one tin!!?'

Naomi replied, mischievously, 'Who buys a set?'

Dad always gets me a bunch of flowers, though! Gradually I have got my own food sorted and cooked for me. One of the

PAs has a butcher who does particularly good sausages. I asked her if she could pick some up for me and she did. Barbara went to ASDA and asked if I wanted anything while she was there. They will bring their own food on duty and can use my facilities. My kitchen is their kitchen. Bizarrely, I developed a habit of eating loads of olives in bed. I'd promise the PAs that I wouldn't choke and they would say, 'You'd better not!' I've also become partial to salty foods.

The PAs are very good at deciding what I'll need for the day. We are much more organised now. I'm lucky to have lovely walks available near my home, without having to get into the van. I will give my PAs ten minutes notice and they can have things ready. A walk down the road involves putting my coat on, getting Mabel's lead out, emptying my leg bag so it is not full when I'm out, locking up and setting off. It works well and everyone is used to what is needed. The pace of traffic past the end of the drive at my family home had been a much more dangerous prospect. My regular walk now is just perfect and much more peaceful. I go down a couple of roads then I'm in the countryside along an accessible lane. It's a lovely short walk which should take around half an hour but by the time I've chatted with a neighbour or two and other familiar faces I meet on the way it's usually twice that long! I'm always meeting people I know down there. The PAs are well-used to chat stops!

Mabel loves it in Davenham! She is my constant, reassuring companion. She still comes everywhere with me and is really good when I am out. I let her off the lead and she stays between the wheelchair and my carer! I don't think she realises when she is on the lead and when not! When I get into my wheelchair, she recognises sounds like the vent alarming and comes straight in. Not for safety reasons but because she thinks she's down for a walk! If I get into the other chair she'll jump up and be properly on my knee which is really funny. If I couldn't have had regular walks with her during the pandemic I'd have gone out of my mind. Mum and Dad often take her for longer walks. Dad's really into his walking. His pace leaves me way behind and I'm getting people asking if I'm alright and need help! I was out once and Dad was way ahead with

Mabel. I was calling her name and a couple of passers-by asked if I'd lost my dog. 'No don't worry. She's with my dad over there, about five miles ahead!'

One day I was walking with another Hannah, who lives near me, and she spotted a Red Fox Labrador. Hannah has a Chocolate one, I've got a White one and Rachel, who I have met regularly on my local walks, has a Black variety and a new puppy which is a Yellow type! That must be a full set between us! We got talking to the lady with the Red Fox. Dad read the details on her badge and we discovered that she worked at Ashton on Mersey School in Greater Manchester. That is a familiar place to me. I told her that we knew someone who taught there. I asked her if she knew my lifelong friend Helen Mitchell. Hannah seemed a little unsure until Dad and I remembered Helen's married name and mentioned it. Suddenly Hannah knew who we were talking about. I said that Helen was a best friend at primary school and Dad was soon proudly telling her about the talks that I'd given to the school, particularly in front of the large audience in the Alex Ferguson Stand at Old Trafford back in 2013. We talked for ages and discovered that Hannah lived in Moulton and was a PE teacher of two years standing at the school. She remembered Helen telling her about me visiting. She was so nice and even knew where I lived! And just to extend the coincidences, her dad worked at my work! I couldn't wait to tell Helen!

I'm just a bit cautious when it gets busy on the walk and there's a particularly tricky bit negotiating a kerb on a sharp corner. Dad let me do it on my own one day because he was taking pictures of my pink poncho which he hates! He sent some out on the family WhatsApp and you can tell from the look on my face that I was not happy with him! He called me a conehead before coming back to my house and going to sleep for two hours on the couch! I went on Houseparty with Mum, Jess and Naomi and he didn't even stir from his slumber! I got Helga, my PA, to hold the phone up and showed him to the rest of the family. Mum couldn't believe it. Him snoring one side, Mabel on the other. Honestly!

Just a few hundred yards away in a different direction is the Blue Bridge over the River Weaver. It is crossed by the busy A556 which runs along the back of my house. From time to time I go down a slope on to the bank of the river underneath. I am confident that I am in control of my wheelchair but I'm just a bit wary of an accident when I'm down there. I suppose that I have become more circumspect with age. How awful it would be if I careered down the hill to the river. We are also concerned about Mabel's safety. She went in after a ball once and struggled to get out. Mum was trying to pull her by her collar but she's quite a weight (Mabel, that is, not Mum!).

I'm able to get to lovely walks in Marbury Park just beyond the Anderton Boat Lift on the edge of Northwich and also round the back of the tip in Northwich. That's been a regular for a lot of years now. It doesn't sound the most romantic of destinations but there are wide, level paths which are ideal for me. I remember watching a murmuration of starlings there. I'd never seen that wonder of nature before. I've definitely got a greater appreciation of my natural surroundings from my dog walks!

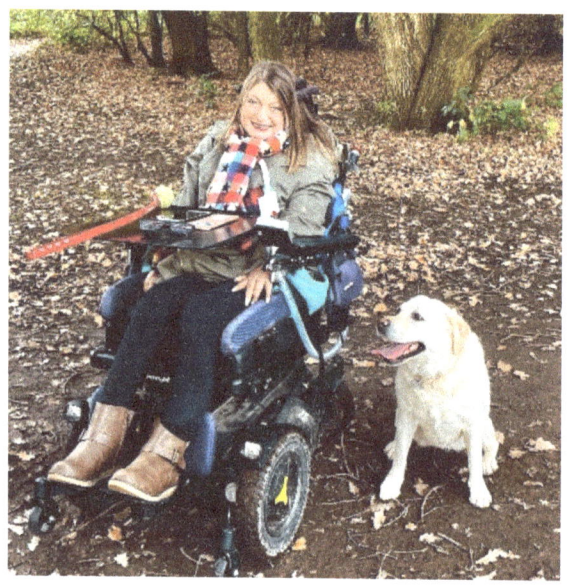

Familiar faces aren't so frequent further away but there are still occasions when we find one. I was in a car park one day after a walk when we met Mum's old boss. 'Lovely to see you, Hannah! Are you doing another book?' she asked.

'Funny you should say that...!' I replied.

An unfamiliar face on the tip walk sparked the most bizarre of conversations. I was with Dad and Mabel. As I was getting out of the car a man walked up,

'Excuse me,' he said, 'is that a breathing machine?'

'Yes, it is,' I replied.

'I thought so,' he continued. 'A friend of mine had one of those.'

'Oh, who was that?'

'Christopher Reeve.'

'Christopher Reeve? Like THE Christopher Reeve?'

'Yes. I went to university with him.'

'WHAT?!'

'Yes, I knew him and whenever I see a breathing apparatus I'm fascinated by it because it reminds me of him.'

We talked for a while. As he walked away, Dad immediately doubted his story. However, he googled the details that the guy had given and they were spot on! You wouldn't expect to meet a friend of Superman's behind the tip in Northwich!

In the words of the theme music to my very favourite programme, 'Neighbours', 'Everybody needs good neighbours'. I've got some fantastic ones in my road. I invited them in for coffee and cake early on. Nearly all of them were able to come and some hadn't met each other before! In my typically worrying way I wondered if they might have been concerned about people coming and going all the time to my house, because I've always needed a lot of visitors for the smooth running of my care package. I needn't have worried. No one has said a thing. I probably didn't appreciate how lovely they were until last year when COVID happened. COVID has had a major bearing on my whole organisation. We started our own WhatsApp group in the neighbourhood. Someone had the idea of us putting a red or green card in our window, to denote if we were either well or needed help. Brilliant! We had cakes on VE Day and I was invited for mulled wine and mince pies at Christmas 2020. I wasn't able to join them on that occasion but it was lovely to be asked, all the same. It was a nice gesture by the organisers, particularly for those on their own.

My first party at the new house was for my 34th birthday in March 2018. I thought it would be fun to have a nineties-themed get together and invited a few friends and family. The Rose sisters dressed as American band Hanson, complete with stunning blond wigs. Naomi took a ribbon from a present from our lovely friend Maurice and put it round Mabel's neck. Mabel even had a blonde wig. Sisters Vicky and Cat came as Patsy and Eddy from 'Absolutely Fabulous', Vicki as Madonna and Lizzy as Britney Spears. Natalie was looking after me that night so joined in as Mel C. I bought nineties food such as Wagon Wheels and Chocolate Dips. We had so much fun.

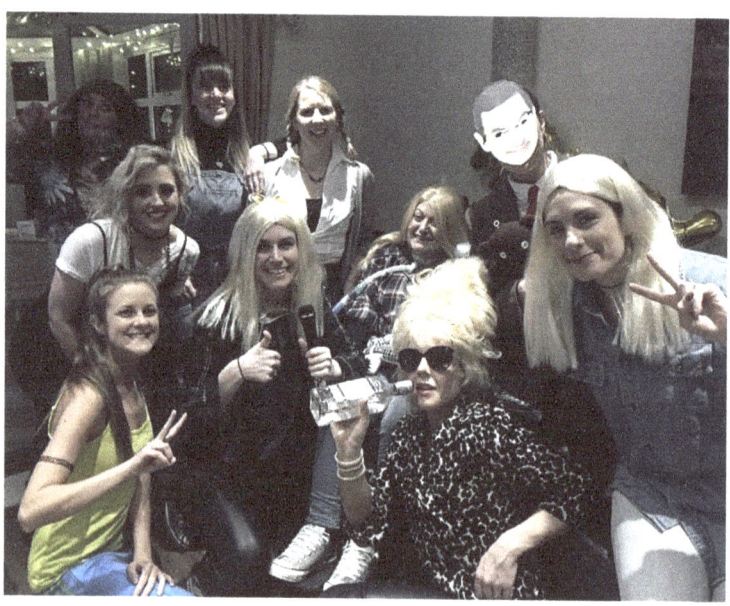

L to R, Cat, Vicki, Natalie, Sarah, Naomi, Lizzie, Hannah, Vicky, Lisa & Jess

CHAPTER TWO

Back In Florida

'this was a holiday when I was to be dogged by health issues'

Nearly a year in to my new life in Davenham I wanted to book a holiday. As you will know if you have read of my previous experiences getting away this can be a mammoth operation logistically, particularly going abroad. However, I needed some sun, hotter and more reliable than that I could soak up in my back garden. I asked about Florida and booked the same place as we had stayed in three years earlier, featured in 'Hannah Moving On'. I booked twelve nights at a decent price. Jess and Naomi were able to come which made it all the more exciting. Steph and Helga came from the PAs.

We flew with Virgin Atlantic again. It was all going smoothly on to the plane. For the first time we could use a hoist but, despite the expectation, it proved trickier to handle than we had hoped. On arrival in America they searched Steph's bag and found a banana in there. She was immediately taken off to a room and we lost her for ages. We had no idea where she was. Dad started to panic and asked loads of people if they could help. It was a relief when Steph suddenly re-appeared further in to the airport and had, apparently, been waiting there for a while. Apparently, you couldn't bring fruit and vegetables into the country!

When we got my chair back from the hold we noticed that it had been damaged and was proving difficult to drive. There was a massive queue of people being held up by us and I felt really sorry for Dad. At times like this I would have been better in my manual chair. We rang Ray, our contact at Permobil in England, and asked him if he could put us in touch with someone in America. A guy came out the very next day and I sat in the sun on a lounger while he tried to fix the problem. As a result, the only thing I couldn't do was tilt the chair backwards and forwards. Dad had to do it.

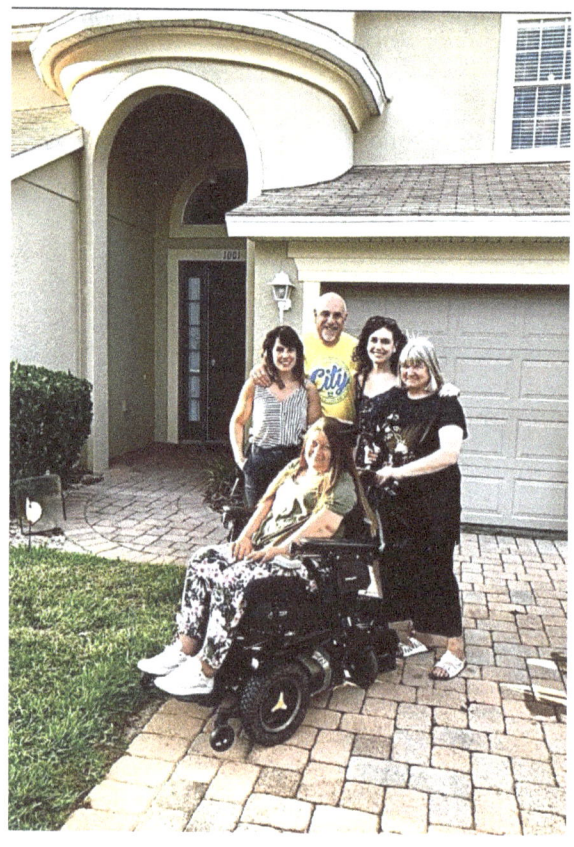

It was lovely to be back at the villa which had given us so many good memories, although this was a holiday when I was to be dogged by health issues. My hair went thinner and I started to lose weight. Despite not feeling a hundred per cent, I was determined to enjoy myself. I particularly wanted to do things that we hadn't been able to do last time round such as Animal Kingdom and Gatorland.

Downtown Kissimmee, just south of Orlando, was one place that I wanted to revisit. It's undeniably tacky but also quirky. We went there on the first evening, before Jess and Naomi arrived, and chose a diner where there was a notice, 'If your visit was swell, ring the bell.' We definitely rang it! Round the corner we came across a fairground where we discovered a funnel cake made of doughnut with cream, ice cream, peanut butter and chocolate sauce. These cakes are popular in America, not least in areas where there are amusement parks. It was so sickly but so nice! My sisters would have loved it.

Next day we visited Bok Tower Gardens, a 250-acre garden and bird sanctuary. The centre piece is the sixty-two metre high Singing Tower which is built on the highest point. Someone in the tower was playing music. The man would come out every now and then to give talks. Bok Tower Gardens was such a beautiful place with so much to look at. I had a watermelon sorbet whilst watching squirrels dashing around.

Jess and Naomi arrived the day after and we went to Gatorland. Mum wasn't bothered so she stayed behind at the villa. It was so good to be back there for the first time since I was eight years old and on my first trip to Florida. We covered a lot of ground that day. Chester was a whopping example of the alligator breed, thirteen and a half foot long and the notice said that he loved eating dogs in Tampa! The Gator Wrestling Show was fun. It was so nice to do what we had done all those years ago, including the obligatory family picture taken inside the Gator's mouth (not Chester's, I should add!). Naomi found a grabber machine and came away with a prize yet again. She is something of an expert.

Epcot was another place that we had been to when young. I had really wanted to go back. There were loads of different countries within the site. In the UK section you could go to Number 10, have fish and chips and visit the pub. In 'Canada' I had scallops. Dad wanted to watch a 360 degree movie but twenty years ago it would have been amazing and now it was one of a number of features looking a bit dated. I couldn't turn easily so the 360 experience wasn't ideal for me. Jess was winding me up by talking about things behind me that I couldn't see. 'Oh my God, look at that!' 'Wow!' She was making me laugh loads but I'm sure other people were wondering why fully grown adults were behaving like this.

On our previous visit Mum and Dad had taken us to 'Norway'. At the bottom of the log flume, trolls jumped out and had really scared us. We were only eight, six and four back then and it was like the worst time of our lives. Going back, we reminisced and Naomi had a picture taken with one of the great big trolls. 'Mexico' was really fun because it was centred around a Disney film that Jess, Naomi and I had watched, called 'Coco'. You could go on a ride and I was able to get into one of the boats which made it more worthwhile. In fact, that was my favourite part of Epcot. In 'Germany' we ate some German food while watching a duck with one leg which entertained us for about an hour! A disabled duck which was coping well. In the 'Italy' section I had an ice cream thinking how nice it would be to be in Italy one day. It would eventually happen but more of that later! I sent Tia, my PA at work, a picture from 'Morocco' because her family are from there. I definitely went round the world that day and, obviously, I had to buy something in every gift shop along the way!

In order to pace ourselves we alternated between a day out and one at our base. Naomi spent some of her time picking up lizards from round the villa. One night a raccoon went past which was very exciting. We hadn't been to 'Animal Kingdom' so had to put that right. There was a safari experience which I was determined to ride on. They hadn't had a wheelchair like mine before but were willing to give it a go. Dad was a bit apprehensive. They warned us to keep our items under control in front of us because if they fell out on to the bumpy terrain we couldn't go after them. This immediately worried me as I had my ventilator. My goodness, it was bumpy and, at times, steep. Naomi was holding on for dear life and I could feel the pressure from Dad's hands on my shoulders as he fought to keep me from falling out. At night I had bruises where people had kept me down. We saw elephants and zebras and I was so glad that we went for it. It showed that there's no point worrying about anything, just do it. For me, it was like going on a roller coaster. I wasn't in control and that made it all the more exhilarating. I hadn't had experiences like that too often. What's the worse that could happen? Going back to get the ventilator out of the lions?! After the ride we watched gorillas eating their own poo for about ten minutes. Naomi and Mum gave up after a while but the other three of us were captivated. It was typical Rose behaviour.

We went back to 'Ovation', a restaurant we had visited and loved in our last Florida trip. The food was gorgeous. Helga bought us doughnuts from 'Dunkin' Doughnuts' as a thank you for inviting her to come.

On the last day we shopped. Mum persuaded Dad to buy her a handbag. The trip was a wonderful mixture of things we hadn't done before and things we had done as children. We got back without major incidents. Dad had researched every single aspect of the trip and given me exactly what I had wanted.

CHAPTER THREE

Another Turn for the Worse

'I was facing the prospect of my life coming to a premature end'

After my initial concerns in Florida, things started going downhill health-wise after I got home. My life post Alder Hey has been characterised by dips in my fortunes and this was to be one of the hardest periods that I had faced. A difficult summer lay ahead of me. At one point I did not even think that I'd come through on the other side. It was that serious. The fact that I did makes it seem not quite so bad looking back but at the time it was horrendous. I was speaking to Naomi and Jess only the other day about the Florida holiday. Naomi remembered how poorly I had been with a sore eye and in bed a lot. I had clearly forgotten some of that.

Mum and Dad had gone back to America for a family wedding and on their return they quickly noticed a deterioration in my health. I needed to have bladder stones removed at Whiston Hospital near Liverpool. My Urology Consultant, Mr Samsudin, worked there. He is just the nicest man ever. Coincidentally, he lives in Hartford, the village where I grew up, and is always bumping into Mum and Dad. I also had a bad pressure sore at this time, just the worst thing to happen to my body. The GP at Danebridge Medical Centre had concerns about me having the operation at that time.

Mr Samsudin told Mum and Dad that I didn't look well but, nevertheless, they went ahead with the operation to remove the stones. While I was in surgery, Mr Samsudin contacted Mr Bell, the plastic surgery expert, and asked him to look at my pressure sore.

I woke up and went back to my room. There were loads of people around me, including Mum and Dad. I still wasn't fully with it but could tell that they looked really upset and that everyone was talking about me. I couldn't respond because when I have had general anaesthetic they have to insert a different tracheostomy tube and it means that I cannot talk. I learned later that Mr Samsudin had spoken to Mum and Dad in the corridor and was very concerned about me. His Dad had just passed away from the effects of a sore. What he had to say gave Mum and Dad a real shock.

The doctors were asking them loads of questions about my care, trying to establish as clear a picture as possible of my situation. It was the most emotional that I'd seen Mum and Dad since Alder Hey. They were both crying. I was desperately trying to communicate but couldn't. It was like a weird and upsetting nightmare and I was so frightened. Apparently, I was lacking potassium, my bloods were wrong and I was deteriorating rapidly. Hospital suggested that I might need feeds to supplement me. Mum and Dad were left alone with me and laid it on thick about how poorly I was and how it had been all too clear to them on their return from New York. They couldn't believe the speed of my deterioration.

'Am I going to die?' I asked them desperately, 'because I don't want to watch you in your life and not be able to join in.'

Jess said, 'You only have that feeling because this is what happened on 'Muppets Christmas Carol'. Jess always knows how to bring me down to earth. I was facing the prospect of my life coming to a premature end, an experience that I had met before.

I was clearly still under the influence of the anaesthetics but from the depths of despondency I had a sudden realisation that maybe I could manage things better, maybe I had been doing too much. It led to some profound thinking and reappraising of my life and was a turning point in my journey. Wasn't it much better to have a shorter but better quality of life than a longer more miserable one? I had been given the biggest fright and really had no idea how ill I had become. What I thought was to be a day in hospital turned out to be a few. They discovered that there was quite a lot of fluid on my lungs and didn't want to release me early. I was anaemic, full of infection and everything was going wrong in my body. Not a pretty situation. I had to have potassium supplements, I had a line put in and intravenous medication.

I had somehow summoned up courage and positivity. For possibly the first time I had convinced myself that I would never concede and give up on my life. I came back to my bungalow on a lovely summer's day and thought, 'I'd miss my house, my dog, my family.' I thought about all the quality experiences that I had in my life. Helga was here and I went through to the back garden where I just burst into tears. The situation that I've got was not of my choosing but I was so lucky to be alive and I wanted to be alive. As long as I have some quality of life I want to be here to enjoy it. It was the biggest realisation ever. I sat in the conservatory telling Dad all this and all the things that gave my life meaning.

I've definitely become more rational about my disability. I know that there will be a time when I don't have the quality of life that I have at the moment but surely that's like any person, isn't it? Growing old brings twinges, niggles and many more serious ailments. I'll know when I've had enough but I don't feel like that now. While I can still get out and about and do things I want to be here enjoying my life. Yes, there will be stressful days which I want to see the back of but that goes for any human being. Nobody's life is perfect, no one is here for ever.

I told my friends about my new approach. I definitely had a new mindset.

CHAPTER FOUR

Rescue in the Car Park

'I found myself sinking deeper and deeper'

After those desperately difficult few weeks I wanted to go away with my friends, somewhere in England this time. I'd looked at Summerfield Farm near Whitby but there wasn't enough space. It was also short notice which ruled some destinations out.

I had come through a period of being very poorly but was still on intravenous medication and needed to take that with me. I found two log cabins with accommodation for ten near Minehead in Somerset and arranged to have two sets of visitors. Anna, Rosanne and Susan could make it out of my friends and they were coming at the start of the week, followed by Vicky and Cat later in the week. It was the first time that I had been away with my friends for ages and ages. Lizzy couldn't get out of school (she is a teacher, not a really slow learner!) and Sarah's grandfather was really ill. Emma and Barbara came from the PAs. It was a long, long drive down and Mabel was amazing considering it was her first trip like that. We went with Emma and Barbara while Mum and Dad went separately.

On arrival there was no bed, hoist, or mattress. They were supposed to have been delivered. This was a big problem and, to make matters worse, we couldn't get hold of the person who should have provided them. My friends were so good, like something off 'Challenge Anneka' which I used to love as a child. They rang round all the local nursing homes and other possibilities to see if any had spare items. We even rang Butlins at Minehead! I got the squishiest, aeriest mattress ever. You can hardly see me in it, as Anna and Susan look on.

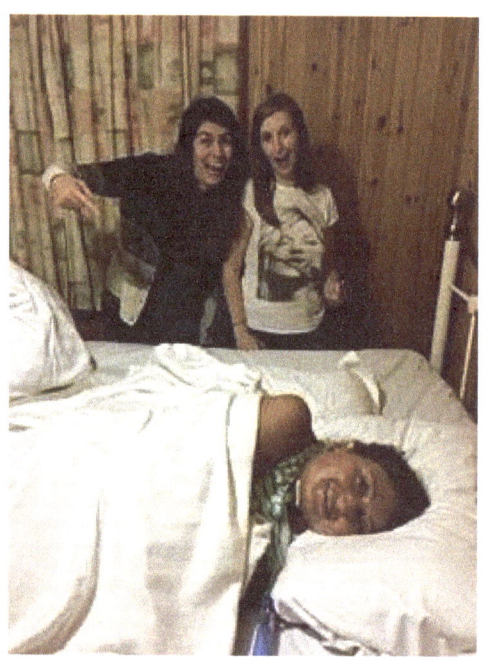

Eventually we got in touch with the guy who had thought we wanted the stuff for the following week, despite my email. He told me he couldn't get it out until tomorrow and was very apologetic. Emma and Barbara and all my friends went the extra mile to get me into bed.

The next day we walked along the seafront at Minehead with Mabel. We sat outside a café drinking hot chocolate and went for a meal at the Hairy Dog. I was able to sit just with my friends, while Mum and Dad sat elsewhere. That was brilliant! Nina behind the bar recommended what to do in Minehead. Back at the house we played a quiz game called Linkee. I love playing games when I'm away.

We all bought kites the next day and took them to the beach. You'd never believe how much fun they can be! I went to the gift shops, as I usually do when away, and had a lovely time. My friends and I went out for a meal in the evening, just us four. They were so good. It was amazing that we could be doing something normal like that. We were horrified to discover that we had left my emergency bag back on the beach! We had been home, got changed and come back out without once thinking about the bag! It was pitch black by now. My friends were so sweet, so worried. Susan and I waited while the others went back and found it! We couldn't believe it when they arrived back triumphantly!

They headed home the following day leaving Mum, Dad and I with some time to ourselves so we went to Dunster Beach just along the coast. It was really quiet but lovely. Mum and I sat next to the car in the car park while Dad threw the ball for Mabel on the beach. We were having such a good time but after a while I suggested we moved on. I edged forward a little then tried to move back but, to my horror, realised that I was stuck in the sand - in the car park! As I responded to various suggestions, I found myself sinking deeper and deeper. Dad got the scraper out of the car to try and edge me out but without any luck.

We tried putting stones under the tyres. A nearby couple were very helpful and stayed on, trying to unpick the problem with us. I was so embarrassed and, to make matters worse, it was starting to get cold. Dad tried to contact a car breakdown company for help, then the fire brigade. About five minutes later a blue flashing light was spotted heading our way. I had my back to the fire engine when Mum and Dad caught sight of it. Their jaws dropped. They couldn't believe it when this massive vehicle drove on to the car park. The friendly couple were still there. They would have a tale to tell! It brought back memories of the time I got stuck in the sand when I went to see the Mitchells at Thornton Cleveleys!

The brigade spoke in broad local accents.

'I'm so sorry, so sorry!!' I said repeatedly.

But they were lovely, saying that they really enjoyed doing this sort of job. I was so grateful to see them. How embarrassing, though! I wasn't even on the beach! They asked if we could put details on their Facebook page. I didn't mind. Dad couldn't believe that I'd asked Mum to put some lip gloss on me before they came, in case there was a photo opportunity!

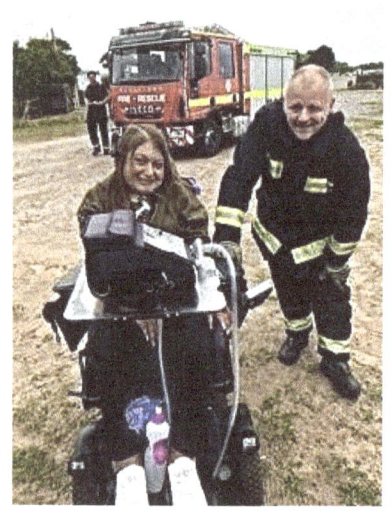

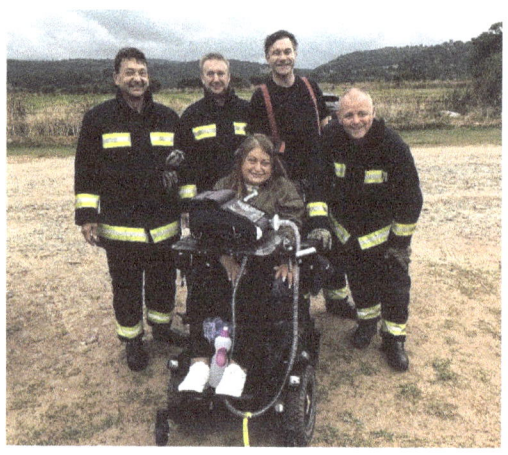

Following the drama, we had a quiet night. I rang Jess and Naomi and told them about the episode.

Vicky Pritchard and her sister Cat came the next day and brought me my IV medications. I was so excited to be on holiday with them. We had a really good time, as this picture shows.

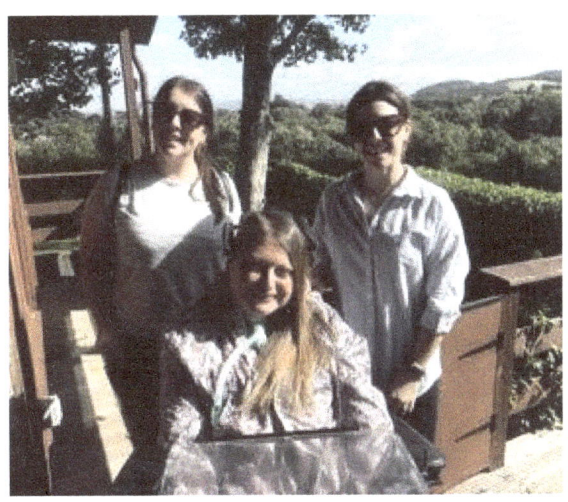

I got a call from the Somerset Gazette,

'Hi! Am I speaking to Hannah? We wanted to write about what happened when you were rescued from the car park.'

'Oh my God!'

I told them that the incident would definitely go into the next book. And it has!

Cat drove the van during their stay, despite not having done it before. We had so much fun, just the three of us. We always do. We drove to Dunster which looked a pretty place on the pictures but we didn't realise how inaccessible the pavements and lanes would be through the village. Poor Vicky and Cat. I was struggling and feeling a little stressed. There was a caravan blocking the whole road as we tried to park. Suddenly we found Mum and Dad who must have had a feeling that we might be in trouble.

On another day we went to the arcades. Mabel hated them. I drove into one of the machines and nearly knocked it over! On the last night we went to a restaurant on the sea front and saw the newspaper with the article in. It sounded very dramatic. Despite that, Minehead had been so much fun.

CHAPTER FIVE

Hannah Rose, News at Ten, Northwich Station

'It was like I was undercover on Panorama!'

I was at work and got a call from Danielle who is involved with marketing in the Leonard Cheshire organisation. When I first came out of hospital and started at university it was Leonard Cheshire who lent me all the equipment that I needed. They have been a huge support for me over the years. I had done a photoshoot at Hartford Station previously for Danielle. She asked if I could do an interview when I got home from work. Sky News wanted to hear about my experiences of train travel.

When I came off the phone I told Nicola and Tia, who were both surprised at the news. I suddenly wasn't so sure that I'd done the right thing in agreeing,

'It's about trains and I don't know much about trains!'

'So why have you agreed to do it?'

'I don't know!'

Tia's housemate used to be a train driver so she said she would talk to her. I wasn't quite sure what help that would be but went with it. I was able to get a reaction from Mum because she had taken me to work that day and I was able to speak to her when I came down from the office at the end of my shift. 'What do you know about trains?' was her reaction.

I had to record the conversation on my phone at four o'clock and send it to Sky. Mum was panicking as she's not technologically savvy. I didn't want my ventilator on because of background noise so Mum turned it off and the alarm was triggered. We couldn't stop it for ages! Then Mum needed the toilet! She was really under pressure!

Despite all that kerfuffle the interview went fine. I've got quite used to such situations over the years. The Sky interviewer asked me about my experience of railways and how I'd been treated on trains. I didn't like to say that I'd only been on one about three times!

The phone rang again. It was Danielle asking if a film crew could arrive tomorrow lunchtime to do a piece for Granada Reports. They wanted to film me at Northwich railway station. I excitedly agreed. Mum said immediately,

'Are you stupid? You haven't even got a car at the moment.'

I'd forgotten that. We had been in Northwich Town Centre near the Seafarer when a car had run over my ramp as I was getting down. It had damaged the end of it. The driver parked up and claimed that she hadn't seen the ramp. My van had to go in for repair and the car which I had been sent as a courtesy vehicle was inaccessible for me. I rang Dad to update him about the filming and he said the same as Mum had.

Barbara and Helga came on shift the next day and I told them where we were going and why. Then there was a phone call from the crew,

'We're on our way but Geraint's going to be a bit late.'

'Geraint?'

Geraint Vincent.'

'But he does the proper news.'

'That's right!'

'Oh, my God!'

I'm a bit of a news nerd and know all the names. I'd watched Geraint Vincent doing loads of news items over the years.

I booked a disabled taxi for twelve o'clock but the crew wanted to film at my house first. I expected the sequence to take a couple of minutes but it took hours because they wanted it filming from different angles. They got a shot of me driving out of the house into the back of a vehicle which not only didn't belong to me but also had doors which we couldn't shut behind me! The driver had put the ramps up. They were the sort which had to be in exactly the right place. As I drove up them he told me that I couldn't go any further because my chair was too heavy for the ramps and was in danger of breaking them. He was particularly unhelpful and I was getting more and more stressed. 'I'm going to die on this ramp,' I thought, yet again. These are the words that I often utter getting in and out of my van. This episode was doing nothing to help that sentiment. I remember joking at Alder Hey about how long it took to get me strapped in and wishing for an automatic lock in the future. I've now got that. I can just drive in and lock into place in a few seconds automatically. Things have definitely improved van-wise.

What would I look like for Geraint? Would I ever get to our meeting? I was only trying to get to the station. We had to ring another car hire company. Fortunately, the next taxi man was so lovely. He asked me where I was going and I explained. His ramps were different but it was hard to get my head inside the top of the taxi. However, he was so helpful. I somehow got in but had to sit sideways.

Geraint was waiting in the car park at the station. I got out with much trepidation. It took me ages. Geraint was so nice. He said, 'I can't believe that we are still doing this issue about the trains. The last time I covered it was with Tanni Grey-Thompson!'

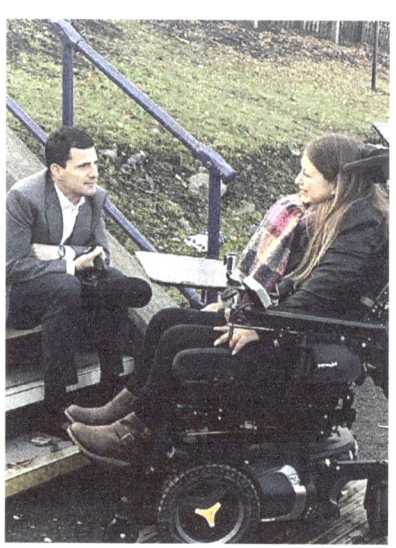

He explained that they were going to put a Go-Pro on my tray. I didn't know what one was but Geraint explained that they didn't have permission to film so I had to look as if I was going to catch a train with Barbara. The Go-Pro would show footage of the platform and I could go to the bottom of the steps which crossed over the platforms to show what they were like for me. They had me looking at a train pulling out of the station, feeling despondent that I couldn't get on it. I didn't realise how good a sad face I was pulling at the time. When the piece aired I got loads of messages saying, 'Great sad face, Hannah!' They thought I looked distraught because I couldn't get on!

Some were also reminding me, 'But you never go on the train!'

'I know!' I replied, 'So people keep telling me!'

I really enjoyed doing all the filming. It was so surreal. Geraint interviewed me at the bottom of the steps going out of the station. In between takes we chatted informally and he asked me about my life. He came across as someone genuinely nice.

As I was leaving the station, I saw a colleague from work,

'Hi Hannah, what you doing here? You going anywhere nice?'

I told her that I was going shopping. It was so embarrassing.

Geraint then wanted some footage at Hartford Station on the main line, including on the train. My immediate thought was having to get in and out of the taxi again. 'I'm not being funny, Geraint, but isn't it all about me not getting on the train!'

When I turned up at Hartford, the taxi found a space but someone who was not disabled had parked in the disabled space next to me. He showed no inclination to move! It was all too much trouble for him. By now the Go-Pro had run out of battery so Geraint used his phone and placed it in front of me. I hid it behind my scarf and coat.

'Drive down to the station,' he told me, 'go into the office and ask if you can get on a Birmingham train.'

It was like I was undercover on Panorama! I asked for my ticket for Birmingham and was told that I had to give notice so that someone could put out the ramps for me.

'Ok. Never mind!' I replied.

And I drove back up the hill to the crew. They were really pleased with what I'd got. We headed to the Coachman across the road for some refreshments. All the chairs were stacked up at the doors so I couldn't get in there either!

Considering that this day was supposed to focus on accessibility I'd not been able to access the car I'd hired, the taxi that came, the space next to my vehicle in the Hartford Station car park and now I couldn't access the pub!

Geraint continued to be really nice and moved all the chairs out of the way. We had a drink as food was not available. We had pictures taken before saying goodbye to the television people. They went into their van in the pub car park and put the film together for the evening news and sent it by satellite. That had been an eventful day! I got home about four o'clock.

I didn't realise that it was going to be on Granada Reports and the national news until someone rang to tell me that she was watching me on television driving into the van which I couldn't use and wasn't mine. I was on the News at Ten as well. Tom Bradby presented it. I love him! Afterwards, people were seeing me in the street and recognising me. I remember doing a choir concert at St John's Church. Someone was behind me and identified me. It became a bit of a standing joke,

'When are you getting on the train, Hannah? What time's it coming?!'

At work, I'd arrive and people would ask me how the train journey into work was. I felt such a fraud!

CHAPTER SIX

A Wedding Guest in Tuscany

'I knew that my long-desired trip to Italy was in the balance'

In the Christmas period after I'd been really poorly my friends came round to my house. Rosanne came with Sam and gave me the most wonderful Christmas present ever. Did I fancy going to their wedding in Italy the following May!? I could not believe what she was saying! Going to Italy had been on my bucket list for ages. Both Jess and Naomi had been and I was desperate to visit as well. Mum and Dad urged against too much excitement at this stage. After all, there were a lot of logistics to sort out and many bridges to cross before then.

However, typical of me, I got on to it straight away. I rang a company called Enable and gave them the wedding venue details in Tuscany. They came back to me with possible accommodation which was only half an hour's distance from where the wedding was going to be held! That was amazing considering how rural Tuscany is. Anna couldn't believe that I had sorted it so quickly for myself, Mum, Dad and Barbara and Emma from my PA team. We decided to go for a week and fly out two days before the wedding, which was on 11th May. This meant that we could go to the pre-wedding day event.

Before then I had another birthday. Now regular readers of my exploits will be aware of my problems with lifts! Well, here's another one coming up. For my 35th birthday I wanted to visit a Portuguese restaurant in Chester. I love meat and they keep serving it on skewers! I had previously been to the same place with my friends and desperately wanted to go again. Liverpool were playing a European game. Naomi and her boyfriend Dan came into Chester early to watch it in a pub.

They lost quite badly and Naomi texted Dad to tell him not to be too hard on Dan about the match. Jess and her husband Stuart went as well. We had a really good night. The meal was lovely. There was a sparkler on a chocolate brownie for my birthday.

The restaurant has an individual platform lift. I've used it before and had already gone up perfectly well on it to the floor where we ate. After the meal I got back on to the platform and, you've guessed it, after my previous experiences with lifts. It wouldn't move. There was quite a big drop below me. I just sat there feeling really stupid. There was a door straight out to the street and it was a draughty place. We were told that an engineer was needed and it could take a while.

Mum and Dad were supplied with chairs and we just had to be patient. We all got hot chocolate and waited in this tiny cubicle for someone to turn up. He came about an hour later and said he didn't know how to fix this type of mechanism. We had to ring Karen, my PA, to say we would be late. They were just about to call the fire brigade (not again!) but had one last go and it released. The place gave us some vouchers valued at £50 but they expired as we weren't able to use them because of the upcoming lockdown! Mum and Dad said they would go back but I didn't particularly want to. It took about two hours to get out in the end and I didn't want to go through that again.

I was really poorly in March and questions started to be asked about whether I could or should travel to Italy. However, I was determined and motivated by the prospect of being there. In my head I was going but deep-down Dad and I both harboured doubts and uncertainties. Fortunately, my health improved and I started to face the prospect that after all my worries I might be getting on a plane and flying to a country that I've always wanted to visit - and for a special friend's wedding! I just could not believe what I might be about to do.

I knew that neither Karen nor Kate could make it. Over the years I had all too often looked at pictures of all the other members of SHARKK (the acronym that my friends Susan, Hannah, Anna, Rosanne, Karen and Kate made up at school) at events without me so it would be a massive deal for me to appear on the wedding pictures this time.

April came and went. We were suddenly in the last few days! None of us knew what to expect. We were excited and apprehensive at the same time. Dad was to be the sole driver over there and nervous about the prospect on roads he wasn't used to, often looking as if they were hanging on a cliff edge. Enable had sorted out everything with easyJet who we hadn't travelled with before. We would travel from Manchester to Pisa.

One of the PAs drove me the short distance to the airport. Mum and Dad went separately. As we met Barbara and Emma at the airport I knew that I was facing a potentially stressful time going through the boarding procedure. We had two suction machines with us and pondered whether we needed them both. We opted for one. We then had to clarify our weight allowance with the travel company. Dad rang them and sorted it fairly quickly. We passed through security where there is always so much to check in our situation. Emma got stopped because she had a lip balm in her bag. We were told we had to pay the extra for the medical stuff. Dad had to clarify with the travel agent that we didn't.

We eventually got to the place where a steward helped me out of my wheelchair to get me on the plane. I was just about to board when Mum ran up looking tearful and red in the face. 'We've lost the suction machine.' She was clearly panicking and we were under pressure to make a decision about our holiday. I just wanted to get on the plane but knew that I couldn't board without the machine. Mum and Dad were in such a stress. I'd never seen them like that.

'What if you were to die on the plane?' they asked me.

I couldn't think rationally but I knew at that moment that my long-desired trip to Italy was hanging in the balance.

They were holding the whole flight up for us. Then a member of the easyJet staff saved the day, going back and finding my machine left behind in the security section! I have never felt relief like that and will always be grateful to the airline for their efforts. And, remember, after we had had the debate in the car park about whether to take one or two, we so nearly had none! On the return journey Mum would sit next to a lady who had been on the aircraft going out. She recalled the panic and was relieved that we hadn't had a repeat drama coming back.

Barbara and Emma kindly slipped me into position so that they were either side of me and I didn't have to flop to one side. I needed something to lie my hands on and one of the stewardesses saw that. She gave me her make-up kit out of her bag which was so lovely of her. I don't think I would have got on that plane had there not been a wedding to go to at the other end.

The duty-free catalogue came round. There was a charm bracelet with an inscription, 'She believed she could so she did.' I have a few things at home with sayings on like that. This bracelet seemed made for me. Mum tried to ignore my pleas but eventually gave me the money. To me, buying this was like a sign and I wore it for the whole holiday.

We disembarked at Pisa, carefully keeping our eye on the suction machine which had become a bit of a running joke by now and was to remain so for the rest of the holiday. At the airport were a group of handsome Italian men. One had a card with 'Rose' written on it so we knew they were for us! They had the van which we were going to use. Mum was quite overwhelmed by them. It was like a scene from the Sopranos. They all helped us to familiarise ourselves with the van.

Dad then had to figure out where we were going. He would do an amazing job getting us around over the next few days. The scenery between the airport and hotel was breathtakingly beautiful. At the same time, certain stretches of road were scary with steep drops.

We had seen pictures of the hotel on the internet but when we arrived it looked more like a conference centre. There was a pool outside. Mum and Dad checked stuff out while we stayed in our vehicle. Our rooms were next to each other with a shared garden. The accommodation was lovely and everything was as it should be. The only downside was that there was no kettle so we had to use a pan to boil water.

We booked the restaurant for eight o'clock. The welcome we got there was fantastic. It was family run and everything about it was just perfect. Through the visit I would practise my Italian on Google and try it with them each evening.

The next day we chilled out ready for the evening event at a restaurant that Sam and Rosanne had hired out for their pre-wedding buffet. I was so excited about seeing my friends in a different country, the first time since I was fourteen and on a school trip. We parked up on this bumpy terrain. You should have seen it! I was so glad that I was using my manual chair. It was the one compromise I had made and it proved worthwhile.

Dad was like a warrior. I will never forget his strength and determination, the same with Mum. A lot of parents would have shied away from the challenge of getting me here to my dream location but the three of us tackled it head on. It was difficult to believe that only two months earlier I had been so poorly. I will be forever grateful to them.

There were already quite a lot of guests present when we arrived, most of whom I didn't know. Rosanne's Mum and Dad couldn't believe that I'd made it! When I got to the table I saw Rosanne and Sam coming towards me. I was bursting with excitement. Next, I saw Susan, Anna and Jim (Anna's husband) coming down the hill. It was just the best feeling to be with them all, in a beautiful foreign country. It's important to remember moments like that when I feel low. It showed that despite my situation I can still have quality experiences. I have achieved some wonderful stuff. When I look back at the many pictures from Italy I just cannot believe that I was there.

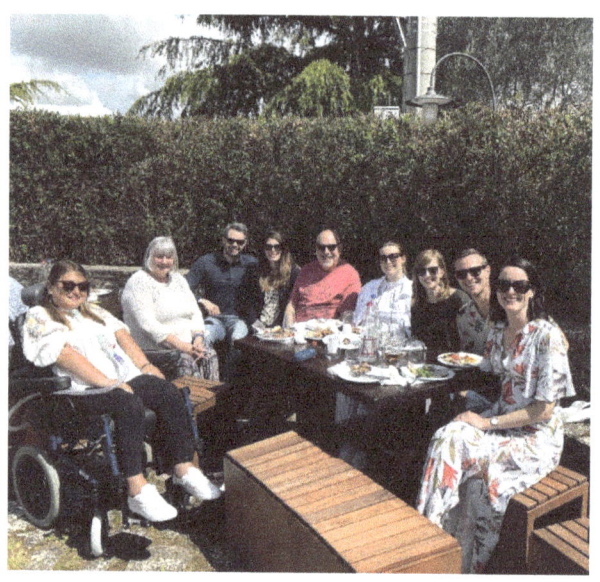

We all sat together. Honestly, it was brilliant. There was a glorious sunset. All I had wanted for years was to get to Italy. I felt like Sandra Bullock in 'While You Were Sleeping', desperate to go to Florence. We left at about half past nine to get a good night's sleep ahead of the big day. Dad drove brilliantly back to the hotel in the dark.

Next morning, I woke up really excited. I'd got my dress ages ago. Barbara and Emma were brilliant at getting me ready. They did my hair and make-up. The wedding was about half an hour away, just past the restaurant where we had met everyone the night before. The service was at two o'clock in the afternoon. When we got there we saw the church on a steep and rocky hill. I didn't know how we were going to get to it at first! Dad had to reverse right up to it.

I got there before my friends. The church was cute and gorgeous outside and in. I sat at the end with a really good view of Rosanne and her bridesmaids as they came in. Mum was next to me, then Anna, Jim and Susan. The service was very much like it would have been in England. Rosanne's cousin sang as the bride and groom walked down the aisle. She had the most gorgeous operatic voice. Rosanne and Sam looked so happy. Her dress was lovely.

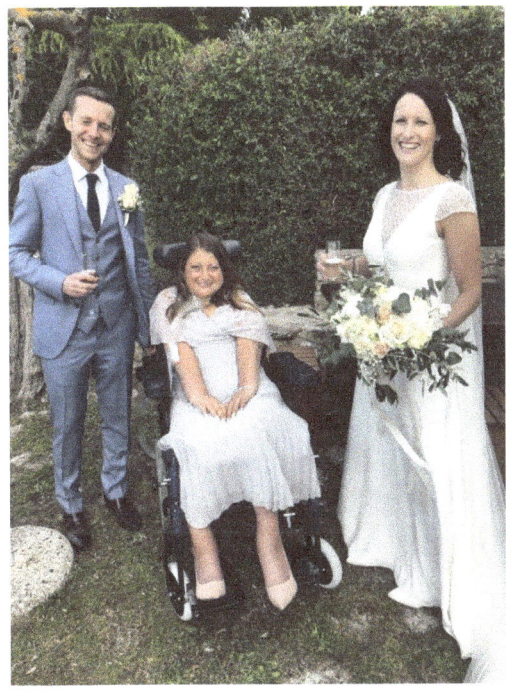

For the umpteenth time I couldn't believe I was there. There were drinks in a courtyard afterwards. Dad had to push me downhill quite a way for that. Then it was on to a delicious looking buffet. The scenery was stunning. There was a musical background which added to the romance. The food was out of this world. It was like something out of a film.

Dad had to negotiate another hill to the main wedding reception. It was at a long table. There were little bottles of olive oil for favours. It started to get a bit chilly. Anna, who was pregnant, went upstairs for some leggings and brought a coat to put round me.

There were so many courses, starting with risotto, followed by pasta. I'd always wanted to be in Italy having a good time. Now I was and my friends were with me! We had the speeches and the first dance. Everything was really good but I felt so sorry for Dad who couldn't drink.

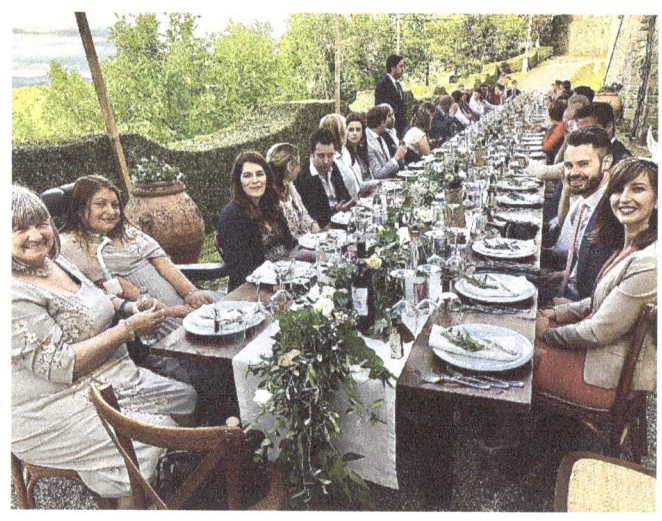

The Rave in the Cave was the title for the dancing part. We stayed quite late but knew that we were going to see them again at lunch time the next day. Everyone was really hung over! They did a massive barbeque for us. There was an actual ice cream van there. We took pictures and I told them it was the first one taken of a multi-generational SHARKK, with Anna already pregnant by then.

It started to rain so we got back into the van. Manchester City were aiming to win the Premier League at Brighton and Dad put it on. The next thing we knew Sam and Rosanne were in the car listening with us! It was the strangest thing ever. I took a video of the occasion and my chair tipped backwards. We were 1-0 down and the Liverpool fans at the wedding were giving us some grief.

We then said a fond goodbye to Rosanne and Sam, who had to go back to the celebrations. When we spoke to Rosanne's sister, she was so grateful that we had got there. There were more tears. Anna and Susan came to the van to say goodbye and Mum got all emotional. However, we knew we were seeing them again in a couple of days' time. We listened to the match on the way back and in the car park at the hotel. In the van, in Tuscany, watching the climax of the Premier League on SkyGo! City won 4-1. They had played a blinder and so had Mum, Dad, Barbara and Emma. I was shattered and tired but we had done it and had a brilliant time.

We still had a few days left to enjoy a beautiful country. I really wanted to go to Siena because it was one of Dad's favourite places. Because it was Susan's last day we decided to go to Florence. Dad was apprehensive after hearing reports of problems getting round the city but had found a useful App to help with finding disabled parking places.

We were near the Ponte Vecchio Bridge which was full of jewellery shops. In the square there was a large merry-go-round. Everyone chipped in to push me round without making it feel like a chore. I was nervous about that chair for that reason so they helped. I had a sandwich which was one of the best I've ever eaten. I was determined to get a handbag on the market. I've never seen so many in my life but found the perfect one. My friends rang to say they had arrived. We met in the square and sat at a nearby restaurant. My friend Sarah had joined us and James, Anna and Jim's old flat mate. It was such a weird experience to be there in that situation. We went through town to a huge food market. I couldn't get in so Sarah, Anna, Susan and I carried on mooching. Then it was time to say goodbye to my friends after a wonderful few days in their company.

I wanted to go to Pisa on the day we were leaving but we didn't have enough time so changed our plans and brought the visit forward. It felt a really long journey. In the car park were loads of people selling things from stalls. My idea of heaven. There was a massive wall hanging with an elephant on it which I loved but couldn't get. I got a few little souvenirs, Leaning

Tower replicas for my sisters and fridge magnets. Honestly, I think I've kept the fridge magnet industry going over the years!

On the way to the Leaning Tower we passed a stall selling umbrellas. 'Seven Euro Umbrellas' the man shouted. They were blue and had different pictures of Italian places on each section. Dad didn't think I needed one but I was desperate to buy and kept pushing, supported by Mum. I even felt sorry for the man selling them! In the end I won and it was one of the best things I have bought. It is still in my van and used a lot. When it comes out we shout, 'Seven Euro Umbrellas!' I'm very protective of it, actually. Honestly, it's the best thing I've ever bought. Barbara, Emma and I bought some scarves. Between us we bought a lot in what Dad called 'the world centre of tat!'

I was excited about seeing the Leaning Tower. It wasn't as I imagined but I don't know what it was I was imagining anyway! We did the usual pictures of pretending to hold the Leaning Tower up. It was funny watching hundreds of people doing the same thing.

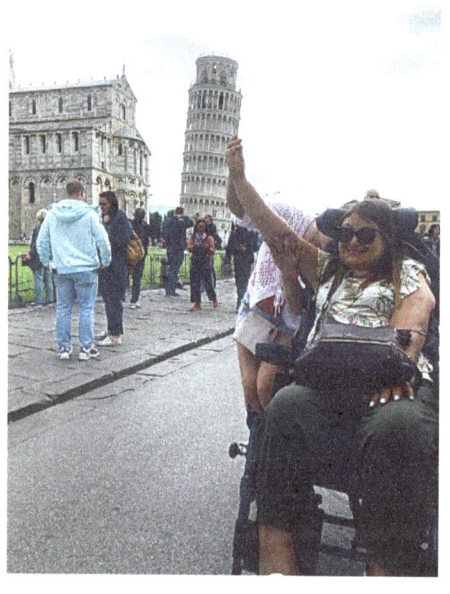

We took loads of photographs and walked round the immediate area. Mum looked for some postcards. The sun came out and we sat out on the marble for a bit. Dad wanted to look at the baptistery. He pushed me in through the exit past loads of people who were letting us through! I couldn't believe what he was doing! It was so embarrassing but an amazing place. He then wanted to go up the tower but nobody else did. There was a long queue anyway! Instead, we went in search of a pizza in Pisa and on the way I got so many freebies such as Pinocchio key rings from stall holders. I bought yet more Pisa-related stuff. Then we headed back to the hotel, probably an hour's journey. I was so excited that I'd seen the Leaning Tower. Back at the hotel I had some amazing pasta and practised more Italian.

The next day we went to Siena. Dad had been to the town a lot with business and was pleased to be there with us. That was really nice. We had a look around the shops. We wanted to get to the centre square but it was too steep so we settled for pictures with the square in the background. We found a One Euro shop in this lovely Italian city! Dad took a picture of me. There was a nun nearby and I had sunglasses on. It looked like I was blind, being pushed by the nun into the One Euroshop! I got an olive bowl and some fridge magnets for Naomi.

On the final night we all had a meal in the hotel restaurant. I had the most gorgeous sliced steak with fried potatoes. The people gave us a bottle of olive oil to take home and we took a picture of us all. They treated us to a limoncello each. The staff urged us to 'come back soon' and gave me a kiss.

It's always an ordeal packing everything up especially when there are so many souvenirs, jars and bottles. Back in Pisa we dropped the van off with the still handsome men and celebrated with a drink in the bar. The whole holiday couldn't have gone better and we didn't want to go home. I know that I exaggerate a lot but this was one of the best times ever. After the drama of the outward journey to Italy we were pleased that the return was uneventful by comparison. I remember once saying to Barbara that I'd never had a sign at an airport with 'Hannah Rose' on it. When I got back to England there was one which she had got

Emily and Lauren, her girls, to make! Barbara and Emma bought Mum and Dad some flowers to say thanks for the holiday.

Mum and Dad took a big risk when many would not have. To be at the wedding and with my friends meant the world. The same friends who had been there at the start of my journey. It was special to be able to tell people who weren't there about it all. Dad made me a photo book. I rang the holiday people to thank them. That was on a Friday, Saturday was an FA Cup match and Sunday was twenty years to the day since I got ill. We had a barbeque with a cake. Lizzy and Chris came round with the twins. It was really fun. Much more about my twenty years later.

CHAPTER SEVEN

Stuck in the Mud

'the car became stationary with its wheels spinning deeper and deeper into the mud!'

I booked the day off work for the annual Cheshire Show in June 2019. I love going there. There's always so much to see, do and buy! Dad and Mum were coming with me. It had been raining heavily up to the day but we decided to chance it. The site at Tabley was only a few miles down the road from my house. It was obvious on arrival that the fields were really muddy but Dad wanted to get as close as possible with us having my chair. A steward indicated that he couldn't go any further than him but Dad chose to ignore his advice and drove on. It wasn't long before the car became stationary with its wheels spinning deeper and deeper into the mud!

'Well done, Dad!' came the chorus. Normally it's never his fault but this time he couldn't squeeze out of taking responsibility! A few seconds later the steward caught up with us and adopted that 'told you so' air. Dad offered no resistance on this occasion,

'I know what you're saying. I don't understand why I drove past you,' was his meek reply.

I did feel a bit sorry for Dad because I know he was only trying to get closer for me. It was clear that we needed to be towed out. After about twenty minutes a van arrived. At this point we were still hopeful of getting into the show. The van driver asked if we had a tow rope. Dad didn't know where it was but, luckily, Mum did and went to look, despite Dad being sceptical. To add insult to injury, Mum found it straight away. She opened a flap at the back of the car and the rope was there! Dad's day was getting worse!

The van's efforts at rescue proved to be in vain. We were stuck too deep. It was suggested that we get a tractor. Well, of all places to need a tractor, Cheshire Show has to be one of the best. It's full of them! We were also told that it might take another hour. By now Dad was posting pictures on Facebook. It was a bit of excitement for him despite him feeling bad about it.

A tractor came and Dad just had to video this as well.

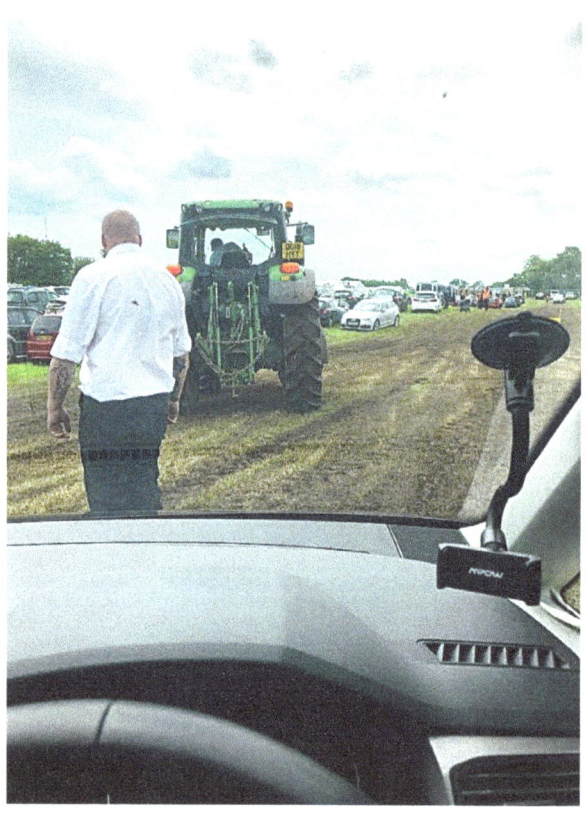

It pulled us out of our embarrassing situation. We drove on but the mud was so sloppy that we knew we couldn't get the chair through it once we had got me out. We were close to a pork pie and fudge stall so we bought some to cheer us up. Then we decided to quit but, before leaving, we went to get our money back as we hadn't even gone into the showground! We were told that it had to go to a panel.

'But we've just given you our money a short while ago and our daughter can't get in. Surely you don't need a panel to sort that out?'

'You are the second person today who has come to me and complained,' said the official.

'What happened to the first?'

'They were complaining because they had flip flops on.'

We decided to go to Fryer's Garden Centre in Knutsford. We had some food there and one of the waitresses was a former pupil of Mum's at Greenbank School. She was really pleased to see Mum. I really felt I needed to buy something to make my rubbish day feel a bit better so I purchased a stone hedgehog! Later, Jess and Naomi rang to ask how the show had been!

CHAPTER EIGHT

Tattoo or not to do?

'Jess said, 'Hannah, just do it.' And it was done on my left wrist.'

I'd been thinking of getting a tattoo for a while. Life's too short and I wanted to seize the day. I thought that I'd get something special to mark my twenty years since the illness overtook me. I wanted to design one myself but just couldn't decide whether to go ahead with it. I went one way, then the other. I looked on the internet for suitable designs. I found one that I liked then rang Jess about it because she had had one done before. I rang the place in Manchester where she had had hers done and made an appointment. Then I wasn't so sure. I'd also been to Knutsford a couple of times but it was difficult finding a tattoo place with good ground floor access. I had tried a couple in Northwich as well. I was going to have it on my wrist on my right arm until the woman in the hospital in Southport broke it. I was with an Occupational Therapist working on getting more comfort in my wheelchair with better arm rests. She overstretched my arm and tried to get my hand to my mouth and my arm cracked. I was in a lot of pain on the way home where my arm was bright red. X-rays revealed a broken elbow. They couldn't plaster the elbow because you have to be able to move the joint. I couldn't believe what had happened. Circumstances had seemed to be conspiring against me.

I was at the Artisan Market in Northwich one day when I saw a notice advertising a new tattoo studio in the town, near the library. There was a girl standing outside and I asked her about it and showed her a picture of the design that I wanted. She said it was possible and also told me that she had a cancellation on Saturday and I booked in!

What had I done?! I didn't have long to dwell on it because, soon after, I got a call from Naomi telling me she had got engaged! When I arrived home, I started thinking about whether I had done the right thing. I'd told Mum and Dad because I needed their help to get into the studio. I also told Jess because I wanted her to come with me when I got it done.

I didn't want to tell the PAs just yet so made up a massive lie! I told Barbara that I was meeting Jess to go to see 'Cats' at the cinema in Northwich at two o'clock. Michaela had driven me to my appointment. Dad and Mum helped me through the door and Jess came soon after. Mum and Dad then left as they were going to watch Manchester City. The girl told me she had worked on the design but that it was bigger than I'd expected. She couldn't put all the detail in it if it was any smaller. My immediate thought was that I didn't want that size but Jess persuaded me otherwise. The lady wanted to know where it was going and I told her inside the wrist. She suggested otherwise and showed me it on the top of my wrist. I really wasn't sure but Jess said, 'Hannah, just do it.' And it was done on my left wrist.

I videoed it being done but still didn't tell anyone when I got home. I knew that Gala was on the late shift and that if she found out she'd tell everyone. I rang Mum and Dad and asked if they could get me into bed earlier. They were in Rusholme having an Indian meal and were due back at about ten o'clock. Mum got me ready quickly, including putting a long-sleeved t-shirt on me. When Gala turned up for her shift she was surprised that I was already in bed, tucked up. Mum said that I'd had an accident with my catheter. We had even put the stuff in the washing machine to cover our tracks.

Gala said, 'Why've you got a long-sleeved t-shirt on? You're always very hot in bed.'

The big reveal eventually came and the PAs couldn't believe I'd done it, asking if it was a transfer. Nobody could believe it but I love it!! In fact it's one of the wildest things I've ever done.

Mum and Dad like it, as do others. Dad had said, 'I don't care what you get as long as you don't get an elephant'!

It is a heart shape in leaves with five roses intertwined within it. Barbara came the next day and asked, 'How was 'Cats'?'

'Oh Barbara, I lied to you.'

'What?!'

I just want this one special tattoo. There won't be any others.

CHAPTER NINE

Lockdown

'it made my disability even harder to deal with'

And then came COVID. Within three months the whole world was facing a unique situation as the virus spread. It would no doubt put many challenges into my already tricky path through life.

It wasn't the best of starts for my family as Dad became very ill with the virus. My birthday in March 2020 had been just before lockdown started and I had made plans to go to a Miller and Carter Steak House but as COVID was picking up speed Dad had suggested not. Instead, I had a Christmas dinner at Mum and Dad's! I think that must have been just a couple of days before Dad was taken ill.

He was determined not to go into hospital and Mum somehow kept the worst from us. Looking back I'm glad that she chose to do it that way. Us five Roses had set up a regular Houseparty chat by then. Dad didn't take part for a week or so and we kept asking Mum how he was. When he finally dragged himself out of bed so that he could make it on screen we knew that it was a special effort on our behalf because Mum told us that he really wasn't well. Knowing what we know now about the virus and the staggering number of people who died from it I'm just so glad that he is still with us. That is not too much of an exaggeration. They were very worrying times.

There was also immense relief that it hadn't affected me or any of my carers because Dad had been around my house only the day before he was taken ill. That was an awful prospect mercifully avoided. I remember him ringing Mum when she was at mine on her own. He used an alternative excuse for calling her so as not to worry us but Mum knew him well enough to realise that this ploy always masked a more serious situation and headed straight home to be with him. We think Mum became ill with COVID as well. She had very bad headaches and the GP said it was more than likely but not certain that she also had the virus.

It was really odd not to see Mum and Dad every day but all credit goes to my team of carers who stepped into the breach and were amazing. Helga and Barbara did my dressings instead of Mum. Various people did my shopping. I got a message from a PA telling me to let her know if Mum, Dad or I needed shopping. That was a lovely gesture. There was always someone willing to take Mabel for a walk if I couldn't.

Among my team there was a feeling that it was nice to have an escape and be able to come to work during COVID. It gave them and myself a feeling that we could get through this terrible situation together, without Mum and Dad's help. It would have been so much more difficult had I still been at the family home.

Then, out of the blue, Mum and Dad arrived unexpectedly at my back gate. They couldn't come any closer at that point but what a lovely surprise it was to see them again after what had seemed like ages.

I couldn't go anywhere because I was immediately told to shield and stay at home. I quickly missed work but Cheshire Police, who had been my employers for thirteen years, were always in touch which meant a lot to me. Mind you, they were probably getting more work done without me there because I have a habit of talking a lot at work! Being off work gave me plenty of time to consider my future there and whether it was now time for me to go down a different career path, possibly doing more motivational speaking. It was a very difficult situation to fully resolve. I have loved all the talks I've given to groups and schools but, equally, work has been so important for my wellbeing and I would definitely miss the people in the office at Winsford were I to leave.

I worried about letting go of something that I'd had for so long and which was precious to me. I'm so proud of what I have achieved with Cheshire Police. At the same time, I recognised that, should I return, I would have to train up another assistant and make different arrangements to get him or her to and from their home. That made me feel nervous. Previously the operation had revolved a lot round Tia, who bore a lot of my issues on days when I wasn't feeling well. Tia was my hands and feet, carrying out a myriad of duties such as cleaning the ball in the mouse I used to get rid of the blusher which came off my cheek! With her just living down the road from the family home where I lived in those early years of work we had soon established a routine to get to and from Winsford. Going forward there would be much more emphasis on my contribution, more flexibility required.

Regular contact with my work colleagues meant so much as the pandemic took hold. They certainly kept me amused during the long weeks at home! They sent me pictures of what they had prepared for lunch as it had been a regular topic of conversation when I was there. I must have a million WhatsApp pictures of lunch boxes full of food! It might not sound amusing to you but the way it developed was hilarious!

Then there was the teddy bear. On my desk at Cheshire Police there is a teddy bear which has been there since Tia and I found it in a box underneath when we moved to it. We couldn't decide whether to call it 'Mansenal' or 'Arcity', both combinations of Arsenal and Manchester City, our favourite football clubs. With the circulation of packed lunch pictures already in full swing, it didn't take long for the bear to get involved. It was now known as Mansel and was taken out and about for photoshoots at everyone's homes! The results were so funny! Nicola sent me pictures of bear driving into Morrisons, on the trolley, then coming back out again with shopping. He had a snack then went speed dating with Nicola's other cuddly toys, then on a date, dressed as a girl with bra and shoes on! There were also some particularly rude examples, unsuitable for re-telling in this book! Bear sunbathed at Stuart's house before going on the trampoline with his daughter. He was on the bed with Stuart's dog. It sounds pretty childish when you read it in black and white but the entertainment was so good and they did it all for me which meant a lot! I could do a separate book on what the bear got up to! Then, one day, in a repetition of what Mum and Dad had done, my work friends were at my back gate with some goodies and the bear! I was nearly crying and it made me realise how much I had been out of the loop. They left the bear with me and it's next to the fish tank in my lounge.

Cheshire Police are very good on wellbeing issues and Babs organised a Skype call with all our team, many of whom were working at home. I told her how thoughtful she had been, doing it on a day and time that suited me. We were on for about half an hour. It was so much fun. Honestly, I had the best time. Hilarious! It took literally two seconds and I was in stitches! It reminded me of what I was missing but also that I was still in their thoughts. 'Work's not the same without you,' one said. Although I missed my colleagues more than anything I consoled myself with the thought that everything wasn't normal for anyone at the moment. I decided that I couldn't resolve the debate in my head as to whether to stay with work or not until we were back to normal.

I felt physically trapped in those early weeks of lockdown and it made my disability even harder to deal with. My friend in Spain said that it would make people understand more what we were going through. Elena lives in Zaragoza. She had broken her neck in a swimming pool accident age 32. Now she's 36. She was in hospital for a year and a half but has found it hard since she came out. Elena had contacted me initially on Facebook, then we spoke on Messenger. She asked how I was coping in the pandemic,

'Do you have aid for 24/7 and carers, Hannah?'
'Yes, and I have nine in my team.'
'Wow, nearly a football team!'
'Can you hold your head up?'
'Yes, I can drive my wheelchair with my head.'
'Have you got any feeling?'
'No,' I replied.

I was missing the live football as were Mum and Dad. Going to the Etihad has always been more than just the football match for me. You will recall how I position myself at a point where celebrities pass by. I will attract their attention, try and get some conversation and, hopefully, a picture. I've done pretty well over the years. Most famous faces turn out to be very, very nice. When they come through I go crazy with excitement!

For years a steward called Alan has helped me attract the names. We have become good friends and there isn't a week goes by when Alan doesn't send me a jokey WhatsApp. He's so lovely. Dad might be missing the football but he doesn't miss me waiting with Alan for a few extra minutes at a time just to see if any more celebs come through. Then his mischievous side will come out. He'll say, 'It's Raheem Sterling.' I'll say, 'Is it?' He'll say, 'No.'

Mind you, my association with Alan did give Dad a moment to savour. The Argentinian full back, Pablo Zabaleta, was coming back to the ground where he had been a fans' favourite for nine years up to 2017. There were loads of people milling around. Alan sorted me out and got me and Dad into a private area for virtually a one-on-one meeting. Alan didn't have to do what he did. I don't think Dad could quite believe what was happening. When I got out everyone was saying, 'Oh my God, I'm so jealous!' I had to have a picture, of course!

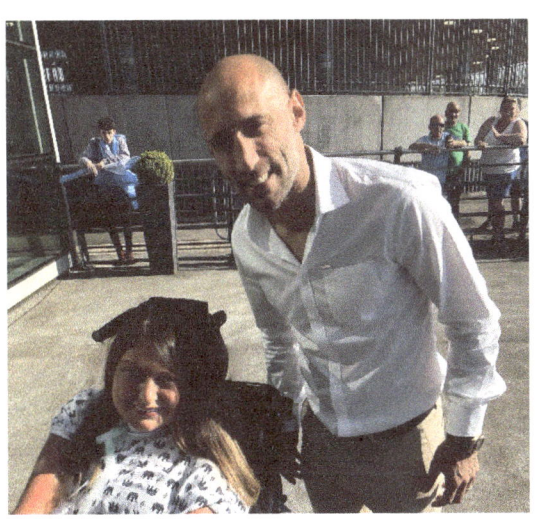

On one occasion last year, Alan asked if I wanted any Tunnel Club passes from people as they left. They started putting them round my neck after Alan requested them. I got some to sign theirs. DJ Mark Ratcliffe came out and I asked him for a picture. 'Nobody ever asks me for a picture,' he said. I got a signed pass from him. I've got about fifteen of them hanging on the mirror in my bedroom. When we have nothing to tie the vent to the chair with they come in useful!

My language over lockdown has become disgusting as tensions over Manchester City have come to the surface. Dad and I were watching them the other week and, honestly, our verbal reactions were terrible, also when City lost to United in the Derby in March 2021. Mum quietly did a jigsaw at the table before asserting that she couldn't manage any longer and went into the other room. When City lost at home to Chelsea in May with that ridiculous Aguero penalty miss I was shouting at the screen and had to apologise to Karen, my PA on shift. I rang Dad,

'Did you watch that? Why were they so rubbish?'

Then Mum rang me to say that Dad had gone to the summer house and wasn't coming out.

'Why have you rung me about that?' I asked.

'Hannah, it's only a game of football,' she added.

'WHAAAT! How can you say that?!!!'

I almost cried tears of joy when Manchester City reached the Champions League Final. It was such big news and made us all happy. I thought of writing to the club to say how much it meant to me and that I'd be forever devastated if they lost. Emma, my cousin, had her wedding arranged for the day of the final but cancelled it for COVID reasons. You couldn't imagine the situation had it clashed. Most of the room would have been City supporters. As it was I watched in the kitchen with Mum at Mum and Dad's, while Dad watched in the lounge, probably because the action was a few seconds ahead. That was so annoying, particularly when he reported the Chelsea goal before it had happened on our screen. At that point he took Mabel out for a walk.

Lockdown gave me ample time to think and reassess my life, too much at times. It was a relief, therefore, to allocate two sessions a week with Sue and Dave and we started this book together. I really looked forward to our regular chats over the phone and I think they did as well! (Too right, Hannah! - Dave) As well as providing material for this book it gave me a chance to put my many random thoughts into words and bounce off others.

Lockdown has made me stress about lots of things. It has given me fearful thoughts about whether I could manage going forward. It has tested my resolve. The inertia has been almost overwhelming. Small setbacks have been magnified. At times like that I've taken a step or two back to the point where I couldn't cope without Mum and Dad again. On one occasion within an icy cold period in January 2021 I fired off my feelings to Jess and Naomi.

Me: I'm so fed up. I've got no one to talk to.

Jess: Ring one of your friends.

Me: I don't want to if I've no reason to.

Jess: I'm going to text your friends now and get them to ring you.

Me: Don't you dare.

Jess: You should really speak to them.

Me: I know but I wouldn't know what to say.

Naomi and Jess have been great and given me brilliant advice but I don't want to ring them all the time or bother Mum and Dad any more than I have to.

CHAPTER TEN

Lockdown Routine

'I watched three successive episodes the other day and it was like the best hour and a bit of my life.'

I suppose that we all settled into routines during lockdown. I was no exception. My daily activity always started with me putting the news on in bed after waking up. I usually got up quite late and washed my hair. My computer would be linked up to my chair and I would come through to the lounge to watch some television. Being a keen follower of current affairs there was plenty to absorb with the daily briefings and blanket coverage of the pandemic. Through Siri I was able, if I wished, to be on my own during the day. If my PAs were unable to hear me I could always ring them.

During the first lockdown the weather was so good that I was able to go out into the back garden. Everything electrical went out with me, including a fan. I got set up in my comfy chair, had a bit of lunch or drank a slush puppy. Then it would be time for 'Neighbours'. I love 'Neighbours'! I watched three successive episodes the other day and it was like the best hour and a bit of my life! You can imagine my despair when news came through in 2022 that Channel Five were axing the programme from its schedule. As my sister Jess said in a Facebook message, somewhat sarcastically,

'Thoughts are with you at this difficult time.'

I once told Nicola from work,

'You know what, my one wish in life would be to go to Ramsay Street.'

She said that I should work that into my next book title. Vicky and Cat showed me a website where you could get a birthday greeting from famous people. I noticed Karl Kennedy from Neighbours, alias Alan Fletcher.

'Oh my God, if I could get that to happen it would be just the best thing ever.'

'Hannah, really?' replied Vicky.

'If I don't get that for my next birthday, I'm going to be very disappointed.'

Following on from that discussion we spent an evening WhatsApping names of the worst celebrities to get a birthday greeting from!

At three 'o' clock I would watch 'Escape to the Country'. From never having any interest in property programmes I have become obsessed. I'd be asking myself way ahead of the programme, 'Wonder where they will be today?' 'Wonder what the budget is?'

It got to the point where if anyone rang me during the programme I'd go, 'No!!! Go away!' It was ridiculous. Sometimes the PAs would be outside giving me a drink as I watched and I'd draw them in to the programme. Next was 'A Place in the Sun'. Out of this programme came a growing wish to have my own holiday home in the foreign sun. As I watched more episodes I started having favourite presenters. Laura Hamilton annoyed me!

Fortunately, I was able to fit walks in if the weather was suitable. It's very frustrating when the rain or cold weather stops me. My walks were very important for me, they still are. If I don't get out, I develop cabin fever. At five o'clock the coronavirus update from Downing Street was required viewing. I never do things by half and it quickly became the next regular obsession. There would be a shift change at six when I would likely come back into the conservatory. A notification would usually come up on Houseparty, 'Naomi Rose is in the house' or 'Jess'. The six o'clock call became a daily occurrence. I had WhatsApped Jess and Naomi at the start of COVID and said that we would have to Houseparty every day during lockdown. Naomi was adamant that we needn't. It happened. Six o'clock every day, although Jess sometimes had to work beyond as 'Pets at Home' were really busy. There was never much to report. When Jess was on she would show us how cute her cats were. I'd tell them about what happened in 'A Place in the Sun' and bore them repeating how I wanted my own place abroad. We played Uno and did quizzes together. A half hour to forty-minute period would contain a lot of meaningless rambling. Here's a typical snatch of conversation,

'What you been up to today?'
'Nothing. You?'
'Same'
'What you having for tea?...Oh, that's nice.'
'OK. Bye!'

We always had to finish by seven as Jess had an evening activity. I enjoyed our chats but it got to the stage where we started to bicker and, as a result, went down to a couple of times a week. Mum was with us on one occasion before suddenly and inexplicably going off screen. I was sure that I heard her answering the front door and her voice saying, 'Oh, hello, I've not seen you in ages.' I was ear-wigging as usual and confused. Next thing she's back on the screen with a bright red face,

'I can't believe what I've just done.'
'Oh my gosh, what now?'

Somehow, she had ended up talking to Jessica Lowe who went to school with our Jess. Mum had just texted the wrong room!

'I was so embarrassed,' Mum said.
'You're embarrassed. How do you think we feel!?'

I get really worried now when she interferes with my phone. I'm never sure where she's going to finish up next!

In the early evening it was time to think about what I wanted for tea. Pre-COVID I watched soaps in the evening and spent time on the computer. Nothing changed in lockdown. Bedtime would be usually quite late. In my situation I just can't make myself comfortable in bed. I have to be put into position. I still sleep on my left side which causes problems because I get a sore shoulder.

I sleep on and off. It varies. Before I was ill I used to sleep so well. I'd sleep on my tummy with my hands under the pillow. I wish I could wriggle into a comfy position like I used to. I have created a problem for myself by watching my phone for long periods before I go to sleep. I should go to bed earlier but during lockdown I've got into a bad routine. I also get second wind sometimes and will talk with the PA on duty until maybe two or three o'clock in the morning. I know that I will feel rubbish the following morning but it is nice to chat, for the PAs as well. It leaves me living in a trance a lot of the time, a strange type of hibernation. I'm often fighting going to sleep. I'll make a strange noise, a kind of snore as the air comes out of my mouth. I will shout the PAs in and by the time they arrive I'm fast asleep again!

I dream an awful lot. Many of them just don't make sense. Sometimes all my PAs are in them but I'm not actually disabled. I'm usually an able-bodied person but with an added sort of stress. I will dream about not getting to the toilet on time. The toilet door might be locked, for instance. One night I was dreaming about Dave telling me that the book could only come in a luminous yellow cover. He had apologised that it was the only shade possible. My previous carers were in my dream as well and I was telling them off.

Having routines has helped get me through each day and week, just like they have for so many others at this time. It's always reassuring when I know that I share something with everyone else. I've had Choir with the Bostock Singers every Tuesday on Zoom. There have been the regular chats for this book with Sue and Dave. I've talked to my sisters every day. Getting up, getting dressed, eating meals, television, going for walks. They have all played their part.

Being without visitors was a pain. I used to look forward to planning visits and the unexpected ones from time to time. I had to be content with life in a bubble alongside Mum, Dad and the PAs but I suppose that enabled me to see more than many were allowed to. Mum and Dad walked to my house quite a lot when we were able to exercise. It took them about half an hour.

It was really good to reach a stage when the government's roadmap was finally relaxed. Typical was the week leading up to Easter 2021 in early April when I had a really nice few days in the sunshine with lots of visitors to my garden. Naomi had Monday off and came to see me. We had a lovely time outside and took Mabel for a walk.

Tuesday was really busy. Aunty Teresa and Uncle Brendan came at half past three and stayed for fish and chips with Mum and I. I spoke to Hughie, their grandson, on video. He was playing on his scooter. Hughie's four and really funny. Some weeks later he came to see me and was so cute. He came in his Manchester City shirt. I can't remember when I had last seen him.

On Wednesday Tara the fire woman came to do an assessment of the house leading to a risk assessment. Nichola did her first shadow shift, followed by a visit from Nicola, my work colleague. We had a lovely catch up and she planned to return soon.

On Thursday I met up with Jess and Naomi at Witton Mill. Dad came as well. We met a lady who had taken in a guide dog which had been abused. Dad got its ball out of the water so thought he was a hero. 'Aren't I good?' We got a Macdonald's from the drive through and had it in the garden.

On Good Friday Mum and Dad came round for a walk. Over Easter weekend Dad and Mum came and we went for another walk. There was a pinboard at the top of my road next to a road sign. It was in a heart shape with the words, 'Don't forget'. Maybe it had been to do with COVID and was going to the tip now. We could only guess.

'I wonder what that was used for?' I said to Mum.

'Well, you put them in your kitchen, Hannah, to attach shopping lists and reminders to.'

'I know what a pinboard is Mum!'

But she carried on explaining all the same.

Dad made afternoon tea with loads of little sandwiches, sausage rolls and black pudding. All the others in the family contributed and we had the food in the garden at Chester Road on Easter Sunday. Mum came to mine on Easter Monday. We went up the lane together with Mabel. It was great to be back to something like normality.

Unfortunately and inevitably, some regular aspects of my life suffered through the pandemic. One unfortunate casualty was our Ronald Macdonald fundraiser which we held annually at Mum and Dad's house each summer. I don't know how we would have got through as a family without Ronald Macdonald House at Alder Hey Hospital. It is a facility that allows families to stay close to their ill children in hospital. Having a base to stay at within the hospital grounds kept some sense of normality for my sisters. Dad could come straight from work in Bootle and we could spend the weekends together. For a number of years we have raised money through competitions, raffles and afternoon tea. The 2019 event had been so successful in beautiful weather and the cause remains a big part of my family's lives.

Many memories of those Alder Hey days are still really clear. Only recently, Mum found loads of postcards that I received when I was in hospital. And I mean loads. There must have been about ten from one of my teachers, Bob Metcalfe. Family and friends sent a lot. The Mitchells wrote about Helen going on the Big One and to a Candy Floss making place. I didn't remember many of the details at the time. In Helen's case that was just as well as I'd have been really jealous! I'd missed out on some really good fun. Others were on the beach soaking up the sun. There was one from the girls on the water sports holiday that I had been unable to go on, saying that they were missing me. A lot of people I didn't even know. I got more out of reading them second hand than at the time.

One night during lockdown I heard a male voice on Granada Reports talking about a lady called Winnie who worked at Alder Hey. My ears pricked up immediately. Winnie was on the ward going from a nurse to a healthcare assistant, dealing with domestic issues. Her husband was on the television talking about her having dementia and being unable to visit her. He was in tears as he spoke. Winnie was just the sweetest lady. I rang

Mum and Dad. They were watching as well and remembered her. One of my PA's went into hospital and someone on the ward was at Alder Hey with me and remembered me. Mum and Dad remembered her as well.

I've just had to do hospital appointments by phone during lockdown. Some of the doctors have been particularly good, squeezing me in when they have space.

I can honestly say that lockdown has not been a totally negative experience. Over the years of my illness I became obsessive about making the most of every minute of every day. Wanting everything to go right in my life undoubtedly added pressure on me to achieve. I would get up early for work a couple of days a week, do a day in the office, come home, maybe do some shopping and take Mabel for a walk. There would be two more early starts when the District Nurses came to do my dressings. I always wanted to make sure that I was up in good time for them. By Friday, I would be shattered. I always wanted to do loads at the weekend then it was back to Monday again. It was a manic existence which, on reflection, exhausted me. Others may have seen that more than I did, particularly Mum who kept telling me that I was trying to do too much. I've even been guilty of going against advice, not staying on my bed when I should have done. Trapped in my body, being on my bed for long periods in the past has been so debilitating. It always makes me go stir crazy.

With the necessary change of lifestyle due to the restrictions I was realising that I didn't need to put pressure on myself to do things every day. As a result, I've had periods of time when I've had loads more energy. A day on, day off approach has made me feel much stronger. By January 2021 my pressure sores were so much better, the best they've ever looked. With Mum (and Dad) not being able to visit for a month the district nurses came in twice a week to dress the sores and Barbara and Helga also did them which was so much more helpful. Staying in bed till lunchtime is not something I'm proud to admit but it has helped me keep pressure off the sores.

Over the years these sores have been the bane of my life. Now I've made a conscious decision to carry on with life even when having them. What's the alternative? I think the nurses have an understanding that for my mental health there's no point me staying on a bed for months at a time hoping they will go away. I'd rather not be here than do that.

After all this good progress I don't want to ruin things. If I've got a day when I'm in my electric wheelchair for a long period I'll be thinking that I need to be careful. When I went to work, I was probably in the chair for ten or eleven hours at a time without being able to find a comfortable alternative. It's only since lockdown that I've really thought about this. I'll have to be back in life at some time in the future and out of the house more, I know that, but for the time being the situation is looking better.

CHAPTER ELEVEN

Zoom!

'The best night ever.'

During lockdown Zoom came into its own and provided endless hours of catching up, amusement and fun. This was no more apparent than in the Murder Mystery Evenings which I held with my friends. In December 2020 Rosanne organised one for Macmillan Cancer Care to make up for us not being able to see each other at Christmas. We each donated money to the cause. It was really good. The storyline involved a doctor found dead in the swimming pool on Captain Crawley-Bumble's cruise ship RMS Whodunnit. I was Beryl Belter, a rising star chanteuse and diva who wanted things right now. Quite like me, to be honest, and I really went all out for it! I ordered a fake cigarette, headband, dangly earrings, pearls and gloves online. I annoyed the carer on duty trying to find the reddest lipstick possible.

There weren't enough people for characters so Anna went from sorting her baby out to playing the chief engineer on the ship, Cyril Slick. This role combined with Lady Iceberg and necessitated quick changes with moustache and wig as she went from East End character to aristocratic lady. Poor Mum had to be involved next to me, continuously scrolling up my phone to keep up with the script. Dad had printed some words out but they were in the wrong order. I properly threw myself into it, talking in a pronounced American accent about Northwich, 'Have you ever seen our wunnerful Salt Museum?', the Manchester derby and many other topics that came to mind. Mum and Dad thought it was hilarious. As for Karen, she seemed to adopt about ten different accents.

After a while Dad went to Lidl. Bearing in mind my storyline it should perhaps have been Macy's. Roger Righthand had cheated on me with dreadfully rich Madame Who-de-Wotwot. At that point Dad walked back in from Lidl with a bunch of flowers! I went off script once again,

'You know what?' I told cheating Rog, 'I don't need you. Look at these lovely flowers that someone has bought me! They are from Lidl, though!'

I ad-libbed so many times that I think everyone was sick of me by the end!

Fran: Hannah played a perfect part. She should be on the stage. It was really lovely to be there and hearing them having so much fun.

Prompted by the success of the evening we embarked on another mystery a couple of months later as well as planning a third just before my birthday in March 2021. I did the second one with Lizzy, Sarah, Anna and a couple of Anna's friends. Once again it was great fun. It was Downturn Abbey themed. I played Lady Flora Rawley, Countess of Grandham. Flora was an American heiress (another chance to flaunt the accent) who has bagged a title and become the richest person in the county. Instructions were to make sure everyone was looked after and keep ordering tea. I could use some of the outfit that I'd used before. My husband had cheated on me (an emerging theme). One was the maid from the servants' quarters. She was played by Sarah who had made a lot of effort to get into the part, dressing convincingly and talking in a rich Yorkshire accent which I had never heard before! Anna was Mrs Pratmore, the cook with rosy cheeks and a rolling pin, also with a Yorkshire accent. It was rude and Mum was next to me, once again, holding things up for me to see. We kept saying, 'Fran, close your ears!'

For the Murder Mystery to celebrate my birthday I was Kylie Invogue in the Smashed Hits Poll Winners Murder. It would be a challenge to keep an Aussie accent up for the night but I picked her because, as you know, I just love Kylie and Neighbours. It helped to make it one of my best birthdays ever. Everyone I asked was able to join - the whole of SHARKK, Lizzy, Sarah, Lizzy's sister Jenny, Celia, Jess, Naomi and my new lovely friend Joanne who I will write about in more detail later in the book. Each of them sorted their own food and drink out. I found preparation a challenge. It took me ages to sort out everyone's character and send the scripts and I worried if they might not like the person that I'd given them. It was quite hard work as I had to save the dialogue in document format then send thirteen lots separately through WhatsApp. Anna gave me some advice, as usual. She is so good at that.

Naomi was Tina Turnaround. I gave Jess Annie Detox with a blonde wig. My friend Katie became an honorary shark for the night and produced one of the best Scottish accents. Sarah was Celine DeLyon, Rosanne was Whitney Housedown. I thought they would like that as they were big fans of each. Kate in Zurich was Katie Shrub but didn't know who Kate Bush was, even though the rest of us did. Karen played Cyndi Leaping under a massive wig with flowers in it. Susan was trying a Brummie accent with a lisp as Toyah. Everyone went to town on the fancy dress. Sarah even dressed her dog as Jon Boney Jovi in a leather coat!

Joanne was Mariah Hairy. We had met through the Back Up Scheme when I acted as her mentor. With her having a range of specific problems we had to work out the logistics of her casting. I spoke to her the week before to see if she wanted to do it. She had one or two concerns and hadn't met my friends. She was worried about going wrong but I told her not to bother about that as she wouldn't be on her own! I didn't want her to feel she had to do it but she was determined. She was in an amateur dramatic group so it interested her. I sent her the PDF of the text and waited for her thoughts on whether she could manage it. She rang me a few times. It would have been easy to give her the part of the detective simply because it was the easiest. I wasn't sure if she would be able to keep a part going all evening because her computer reads each piece out. She expressed a preference for another character, not the detective. She became Mariah Hairy.

Mum and Dad watched the first five minutes. They wanted to see everyone and I wanted them to. Sharon, my PA, helped me. It was lovely to have everyone involved. Before we went to characters each introduced themselves to Joanne, who had requested it. Afterwards she sent me a text saying it hadn't put her off doing it again. There was ad-libbing, improvisation, hilarity and plenty of chat afterwards. I was nearly crying by the end. It was so emotional. What an effort they all put in and Joanne was there and was so good. It was the best night ever. Naomi was so funny as Tina. We asked her to do a dance at one point but she refused as she had pyjamas on the bottom half. Karen said she sounded more like Mr T!

I was a glutton for punishment having already booked yet another Murder Mystery for my birthday the next day with Mum, Dad, Jess, Stuart, Naomi and Dan. Overnight Naomi sent me a picture of Pep Guardiola with his head in his hands alongside the caption, 'Oh no, not another Murder Mystery!'

'Murder on the Dance Floor' preceded a Christmas Dinner which I had requested from Dad for my birthday. We had eight characters and seven people so Jess suggested her friend Candy. The organisation was much easier this time round. I was ready and up for it again. If anyone needs me to do one now, I'm on it. Dad wore a Rastafarian wig for the character of Baron Hardnose. Ridiculous. Mum was Darcey Bussell. Dan wore a train driver's hat. It was really good fun.

Previously, Jess and Naomi had given me a pretty bracelet as a birthday present and told me that my second part was following later. After the Murder Mystery had finished, Jess asked if someone could share the screen. Jess sent me a video on WhatsApp. It was the funniest thing ever! Karl Kennedy from Neighbours was sending me a message and birthday greetings!

'I know you're a lifelong Neighbours fan. Thanks so so much for that. Jessica tells me that Neighbours has been a bit of a lifeline for you during lockdown... It's been a very tough year for you and you deserve a very special birthday.'

I was made up about it, totally in shock! The next morning, I woke up and there was a WhatsApp from SHARKK saying 'G'Day birthday girl' (me having been Kylie in the Murder Mystery). I said 'Just wait till you've seen my present!'

'Is it a cut out of Jason Donovan?'

'Even better!'

I sent them Jess's video and they couldn't believe it.

There was a video from the girlies from work. (Vicky P, Cat and Vicky B). It was Karl again! I couldn't believe that they had had the same idea as Jess. It was hilarious! The messages were so different.

'I hear you are a huge fan of Neighbours and you don't mind Dr Karl. You sound incredible and I'd love to meet you. Because you love Neighbours it makes me perfectly qualified to wish you a very very Happy Birthday... Apparently, you've done a bit of TV yourself, on train stations. Not quite sure what that means but it sounds very very interesting. Have a fantastic birthday and thanks for watching Neighbours. Cheers!'

Jess, typically, said,

'Karl will be quids in after that. They are probably the only two he'll have done.'

It was a while before I could thank Vicky, Cat and Vicki face to face but we had a lovely catch up when they came round to mine. I told them I couldn't believe what they had done.

My friends and I have used Zoom such a lot. It's not just been about Murder Mysteries! We had a virtual baby shower for Rosanne at the height of lockdown in April 2020. It was a boiling day and I was in the back garden. Karen was on from Barcelona, sitting on her balcony in a bikini. Kate was in Zurich. We sent in pictures of ourselves for 'Guess the Baby?' and made little rosettes with Aunty Hannah etc on.

On another occasion Anna made up a quiz. We all sent our pictures and had to guess who was who. We made cakes and biscuits. We've done some really good quizzes.

We did an Escape Room through Zoom for all my friends to celebrate Lizzy's birthday. On this occasion I found it really hard and just sat, letting the conversation swim past me. At one stage Sarah asked me if my screen had frozen! I must have barely moved! I WhatsApped Anna separately and told her that I was really fed up. On Sunday we had a really long chat. I told her how hard it was being unable to move and it felt like I was going to explode. I didn't know what to do. Anna's so good, the voice of reason. She told me that she had had a difficult time during the pandemic. I felt much better for the conversation.

Prior to Naomi's wedding I linked with Jess and Lisa, the other bridesmaids, in secret to organise a hen do. Lisa was doing the organisation for the hen party. She was chief bridesmaid and used a spread sheet. She put Jessica and I to shame with her organisational skills. I had got to order things for games but with Amazon Prime I could leave it till nearer the day. There was no point in cluttering up the house.

Zoom kept me in contact with the Bostock Choir if I was feeling well enough to participate. In July 2021 the choir finally met up again face-to-face. It was at the Yew Tree Inn in Bunbury. We all had a meal then sang together, with appropriate space between us. It was amazing to hear everyone together after months online. Mum sent a three-minute video of my lap. I had promised the choir some video but didn't expect that!

CHAPTER TWELVE

A Welcome Break by the Sea

It was one of the funniest pictures ever and remains one of my favourites.

With 2020 having been such a difficult year for all of us I once again reached a point where I needed to have a break from it all. Normally, I would have been looking at the Canary Islands or Spain, somewhere with lots of hot sun, but knew that my horizons were limited because of COVID restrictions. We had already missed a planned trip to Lanzarote which was a bit rubbish.

By the summer I was really fed up at not being able to get away somewhere. I'd had a good look at places in England but nothing had been organised as yet. I couldn't get out much. Everything was getting on top of me. The pressure kept building and building inside me until one night at Mum and Dad's I got really upset and let it all out. I just couldn't stop crying. I needed that break so badly and it was so important that I had all five of us Roses there although I didn't think Jess would be able to go anywhere with us. She lived and worked in Manchester where the situation was really bad.

I got obsessive about a holiday. My specific requirements ruled out a lot of places. I really wanted to go back to Minehead, where I was probably a minor local celebrity by now, but they didn't have enough space in the accommodation we had used. Summerfield Farm near Whitby came up and there were also possibilities in Bridlington, further down the Yorkshire coast. I rang Sue and Dave and they just happened to be walking nearby at Anderton Boat Lift so they came round and helped me choose with their experience of places in Yorkshire. Summerfield Farm it was to be and Jess and Naomi were both able to join us. I would love to have taken Stuart and Dan as well but they didn't have enough room. Dad told me to just book it and we settled for the end of September 2020. I let the PAs know of my plans and asked if any wanted to come. I took Barbara and Emma. They should have been going to Lanzarote so it made sense to have them there.

There was already a bed and a hoist available in the accommodation so I just took my own mattress. Jess and Naomi arranged to meet us there. Jess brought my manual wheelchair which proved to be really helpful. The place was lovely and I was really excited about being away from home. We went to B & Ms for supplies and there was an Aldi and a Sainsburys nearby so that was really handy.

Whitby was only a few minutes away and it was really windy when we made our first visit into town, as the picture on the front cover shows! It was a Saturday. We looked at gift shops, of course, taking care to observe the social distancing rules. It was really busy and it was a good job I was in my manual wheelchair. It started raining and Naomi pushed me into the doorway of an arcade. When we came out Jess took a great picture of us all wrapped up and in masks. I couldn't see a thing through my glasses! It was one of the funniest pictures ever and remains one of my favourites. We ended up in the Co-op of all places. Back at the cottage we put the fire on and warmed up. Dad brought some fish and chips back from Trenchers, after a recommendation from our friend Sheila Snowdon! They were the best I'd ever tasted! I'd bought some cakes for Jess and Naomi. We all chatted away and it was really nice.

The next day we went down the coast to Scarborough. I particularly wanted to go to the Sea Life Centre. Nobody else was excited about the prospect but they gave in to me! It was to cost us about a hundred pounds! Someone handed Jess a parking ticket which still had time left on it and said, 'You won't be in there long, love.' He was right. Hardly anything was open. There were just some otters, penguins and some seals. Then we went into the tunnel where all the fish were. Nobody had told us how inaccessible this was. By the time we got to the end there was a great big queue behind us. Wheelchair users had to turn round and return along the way we had come in. What a nightmare that was!

When we came out, Jess and Naomi were eager to point out that they had been proved right, 'Told you! Told you!' they taunted me playfully. We parked in an underground park on the seafront. A car alarm sounded. Jess said, 'Who's let that happen? That's so annoying.' It was actually her car! She had locked Naomi inside it! When we got her out she kept going on about being traumatised and claustrophobic. We went to a fish and chip shop to raise her spirits. There was a lift up one floor and, despite many previous problems over the years, I managed to negotiate this one with ease. My eyes are often bigger than my stomach and I ordered a fish platter, not realising the size of it. Dad said, 'Don't think you are leaving any of that!' However, I had to and Mum, Dad and I finished up having it for tea that night. The waitress who served us was really lovely. A group of teenagers came in and ordered large fish, chips and rounds of bread and butter. When the waitress brought it over they said, 'We're not hungry any more' and walked out! I felt really sorry for her.

Back on the prom I saw some of those grabber machines. There were sloths inside and I really wanted one because I've got a thing about them. Naomi is so good at winning things on these and offered to have a go. She hooked one first time! There was a fortune teller machine like some I've used before. Whenever I see one I'm always tempted to have a go. When the card came out, it read, 'You will have some good things delivered when you get home.' Everyone howled because there's barely a day goes by when I don't get a parcel delivered!

Jess and Naomi left that evening, taking my manual chair back with them. It had been so useful. We had had such a lovely time together.

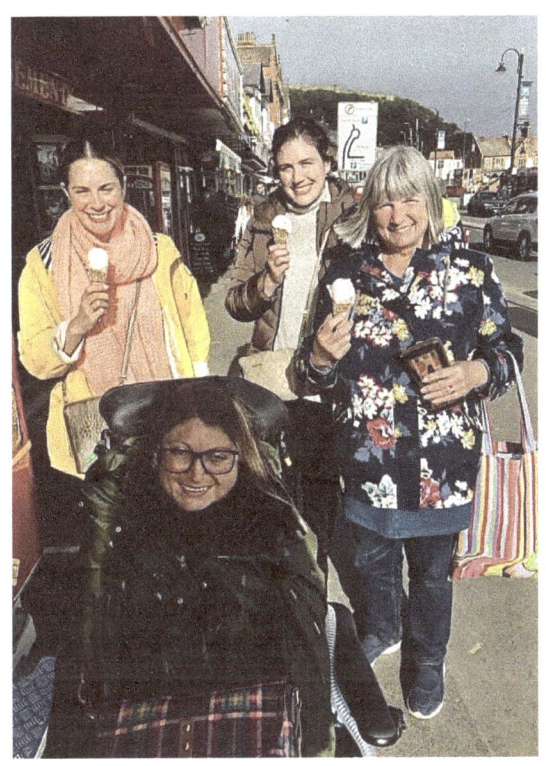

Next day we headed to the indoor market in Scarborough. It had looked good on the website but when I got there it wasn't!

We decided to try Bridlington. We knew that Barbara and Emma were going so we had asked them to let us know if it was worth a visit or not. By the time they rang that it wasn't, we had arrived! There was a lot of work being done on the sea front so it wasn't an ideal day to be going. Back in Scarborough I took Mabel for a really long walk. The waves were really high and it was enjoyable. After a hot chocolate we went to Peasholm Park and didn't realise that it was where Dad had visited in his childhood. Grandma and Grandpa used to take him to see the model ships enacting battles on the lake in the summer. I loved it there and it was great for Mabel, too. It is one place that I really want to go back to.

We had a meal at the nearby Hare and Hounds. I had checked it out on Google, looked at disabled access and booked a table. The door proved trickier than I thought but I had a lovely pie and as we were eating there was a playlist on which featured all my favourite songs from the nineties, including Robbie Williams. I kept saying, 'I love this song, I love this song...'

We had one last trip into Whitby before we left for home. I crossed the river, bounced up and down along the cobbled area in my electric chair right up to the Abbey with Emma and Mum. I wanted some jewellery to remember the trip by and there was this market stall but I couldn't get over a step. Some people tried to help me and were very kind. A woman showed me a bracelet and I told her I'd buy it. I've never had much resistance where shopping is concerned! Then she pulled out a beautiful bracelet with a Tree of Life on it. She told me that she wanted me to have it. That was so lovely of her.

We bought scampi and chips from the Magpie Cafe by the harbour and ate it whilst sitting on a bench. I told Mum and Dad that I really wanted to come back on my birthday. I looked down at the newspaper inside the scampi box and, would you believe it, my birthday date was written in the corner! A sign, surely?! On the way back to the car Mum and Dad met some friends, parents of one of Jess's friends. I couldn't believe it as we were so far from home.

The trip did me the world of good. Everyone had a great time and were so good to me, as well as giving me the usual stick! This included working out my three most annoying habits!

3   When I talk to Siri on the phone (they shouldn't be upset because it saves them a job)
2   When I start on a topic then go off at a tangent
1   When I make a noise to make Mabel bring me a toy

Mabel was so good on the holiday, by the way. She couldn't go into Sea Life (so didn't miss much there!) but went everywhere else.

CHAPTER THIRTEEN

A Brilliant Family Christmas

Health-wise, I felt the best that I have for years

Despite all the doom and gloom felt around the country and the many restrictions announced by Boris regarding celebrations for 2020 I was to have such a good time at Christmas. I've always been a big fan of the festive season and having the best tree ever was a great tonic. Unfortunately, no one could come and see it which was so annoying as I desperately wanted to share my joy with others in my own house at the end of a year when Dad had been so ill.

I have always clicked into festive gear well before Christmas Day. This year I bought loads of cheeses at the Artisan Market in Northwich. They were on offer. Four for £10. I also chose my own Christmas present, a picture which I wanted for my hall, and a jumper that I didn't really need! Typical of me! I was so excited to go back to the market after lockdown. I was a bit nervous about how busy it would be but the weather had put a lot of people off. It was nice to see some of the stallholders who I knew such as the clothes lady, the shoes lady and the pie lady,

'Hi, how are you doing?' they all asked.

I was looking at the earrings and wanted to buy two pairs. A familiar woman's voice behind me suggested that I didn't need two pairs. It was Mum. She agreed to meet me at the car and I went back to get the other pair. The woman was surprised,

'Didn't your Mum say you didn't need two pairs?

Yes, but I am 37 years old.'

For some years Dad has been involved with Rotary Club and it has been his habit to dress as Father Christmas and tour the streets around the Northwich area. This year he had to resort to good old Zoom. He sat in position, just needing to dress as

Father Christmas on the top half of his body. One day, a little girl asked how many deer he had and he had literally no 'ideer'! He was asked to name them,

'I can't. There's just too many,' was his answer.

Dad describes it as the weirdest thing he's ever done, talking to children on the internet when they are asked not to speak to strangers. Here he was - a Jewish Father Christmas.

Stuart and Dan joined us for the first time. We were so lucky to be able to do it that way because so many of my friends weren't able to get together with families because of restrictions. We all went for a COVID test in advance of the day and didn't go anywhere for four days after. I put pictures on Facebook but wanted people to know the background. We were being very careful but it was still a strange experience after remaining at distance for so long.

I got to Mum and Dad's about half past eleven. We had a brunch round the table followed by presents. Having spent much of the previous month in his outfit, Dad still insisted on getting dressed as Father Christmas to give out the presents! It was quite a surprise when he came downstairs. Mabel went nuts!

Naomi was actually my Secret Santa but I couldn't resist buying the present which I gave Jess. It was a calendar with cats pooing on it. Not the sort you would normally see on sale in the Garden Centre!

Mum and Dad had made a book of my House of Commons experiences, described in 'Hannah Moving On', including the Tweets connected with it. It was really nice and a lovely surprise although all I seemed to say when I looked through the pages was, 'Look how fat I am.'

My present from Naomi was so unusual. It was a Barbie in a wheelchair! We had so many laughs out of it. It got pride of place in my house and we are going to get a little ventilator, maybe a little Mabel to go with it. I had quite a lot of presents to open from PAs and friends but Naomi gets so impatient as she opens them and rushes me through.

There were loads of funny moments. Stuart wrapped the presents for Jess and she was going mad because he'd left them in the Amazon boxes! He said it saved on filling the bin. Mum managed to record the whole hour and a half of present opening by accident. Gripping stuff!

We watched a classic Top of the Pops as Dad did the cooking. He is an amazing cook and attributes this to his mother, Grandma Ruth. It was an incredible meal. Jess prepared the sprouts, a traditional part of our family Christmas. I've never seen her so enthusiastic about crackers. They were from Marks and Spencers and the gifts were really useful. She got some new measuring spoons and I got something to put in the pan when you are boiling an egg.

There were good-natured insults flying around all day and absolutely no respect for the eldest sister in the family. Good job that I can take it! Team games created much amusement and competition. We played 'Tension' where you had to list the top ten of, say, Tom Cruise films. Jessica has never grown out of being a bad loser. She gets really mad. I didn't like the fact that teams were helping each other. It definitely caused tension for me.

As always, we played 'Pass the Sprout' which is a variation on 'Pass the Parcel'. It says suitable for children from age 3 on the packaging. That just about sums us up. Mum's responsible for buying it each year, the sprout being a tissue-wrapped ball. We got it from a different outlet this time and it was a bit rubbish, to be honest. The prize was two crayons. A few rounds before Dad had got a picture to colour in so that's probably why it was such a random prize. A joke session followed but I'm useless at telling them.

Health-wise, I felt the best that I have for years at Christmas. Not being together often enough in the previous months made it all the better. Everyone was really relaxed. I didn't want the day to end and finally left around eleven after a day when we had briefly managed to forget COVID. That felt so good! I was able to hear a lot of it again because, as a result of forgetting to press 'Stop' on my phone, I found an hour and more of small talk, not always stuff I'd want other people to hear!

By comparison, Boxing Day was quiet and I spent it with Mum and Dad. We watched a film and ate leftovers from Christmas dinner, bits of all three courses. I always like that the day after. There were a couple of turkey pies as well which I ate over the next few days.

A brilliant birthday followed a brilliant Christmas. The entertaining Murder Mysteries that I've already spoken about were just part of one of my best birthdays ever, a surprising thing to admit when the day occurred during a time of restriction. I had loads of lovely messages on Facebook, hearing from people as far back as Alder Hey Hospital. This is when Facebook is at its best. Everyone thought that my Neighbours videos were hilarious. I got a WhatsApp from Clare down the Close,

'Happy belated. Ps so good to know there's another cheeky Neighbours fan on the street! When should we re-name our road Ramsay Street?! Maybe for the day of the biggest BBQ ever post-pandemic!'

The birthday day was lovely and sunny. I couldn't believe it! Mum's friend Caroline bought me a lovely plant. Caroline used to be a carer, now she is in the Book Group that Mum is a member of. Mum bought a Happy Meal which I ate at the front of the house. There were flowers from Mo, my hairdresser, and Stephen Bartley. The Bartley family have always sent flowers even though Mum Krystina sadly passed away in 2020. I was at school with their children. Long-time friend Maurice dropped by. I caught up with others on the phone and met loads of people on my daily walk.

It was good to get into my comfy chair. Dad had come away from work early. My friends were really kind. Sarah had made Brownies with salted pretzels inside and embroidered a cushion with an elephant on the front. It was beautiful. I got a throw with Mabel's face all over and money from my PAs. Anna took a picture of the Davenport Teas and WhatsApped, 'Happy Birthday Han. Would you like to join me in your garden for afternoon tea after it's all over?' Lizzy's twins sent a card. Loads of cards arrived including one from the postcode lottery of all places. Even Simon, my long-standing ventilator technician from Southport, sent me an email.

All in all, the attention made me feel that I was one very lucky person.

CHAPTER FOURTEEN

Managing my Team

'I'd give anything to be on my own for just a day.'

I have had a team around me since leaving hospital but it is interesting to think back and see how the management has changed over the years as challenges have presented themselves. I have always tried to ensure that everyone is familiar with the system and knows their roles but there's no doubt that the pandemic has thrown up its own individual challenges. I've been so lucky not to have needed a new member of staff during lockdown because we couldn't have offered training.

Training has been a regular aspect throughout, both for myself and my team. I've been doing some employer training on Zoom which has been really practical. It made me really think about my situation. The down side was that it has been heavy going at times. It was about three hours long and the first time I've had access to this sort of support. I involved Janet into it as well. She is my former Maths teacher who has been such an important part of my team for years now. I think it started from something connected with my friend Sarah. Janet came to help me out and now runs the logistics side of the operation – payroll, annual leave and rotas. I have praised her many times before and still don't know what I'd do without her. Janet is so efficient, caring and good-hearted. At school she was really strict! I know that I can call her at any time if I am upset or need help. She's only two minutes away. She'll explain in an interview with a prospective PA that she used to teach me and I still think it sounds really weird. Janet will do anything for anyone. We go out for lunch with Mum and Mum's old friend, Sue Daly. Sue is lovely. Mum and Sue used to teach together.

Sue also knows Janet. Sue and Janet work at St Luke's Hospice in Winsford, a charity organisation. Sue's always sending me things through Janet which she thinks I'd like.

The lady running the training wanted to know when I first employed PAs and what it was like before they worked for me. Those who didn't come from the old family home with me can't believe what it used to be like, being round a family all the time. Now they've got their own room and better facilities.

I used another Employer Training session as a counselling session. It didn't start well because I couldn't get into the meeting! I just couldn't find the link. The instructor was sitting for about twenty minutes waiting for me! Eventually we got going and I explained what was stressing me out. She asked for examples and gave me practical techniques on how to overcome them. I have learnt some good advice about situations like that. As an example, I have been encouraged to say, 'I can't answer you at the moment, can I get back to you?' instead of getting involved too much too soon. Better to wait and react in a considered way.

Simon has been been coming regularly to service my ventilator and to do training for the PAs on the ventilator, including an update on the mechanics of it. There has to be a refresher every year, paid for by the health authority, and on demand. Simon has always been on the end of a phone, someone who you can trust and who knows his stuff. He has now retired. I will miss him because he has been, to quote an overused modern expression, such a big part of my journey. He has worked in Southport at the Spinal Unit for twenty-five years. When I first became ill I should have gone there but there wasn't room. A consultant came to me to assess the damage and talk to Mum and Dad. When I got to the adult care situation Southport Spinal Unit took over my ventilation from Alder Hey.

My final visit from him was in February 2020. Simon did a training session with six PAs and it was so good to have them together in lockdown and hear the laughter coming from the next room. I gave him a bottle of whisky and a card. It was a sad visit and I felt weird after he had gone. He came with his replacement, Gary, who is also very nice. I've met Gary before. He stood there while I went on to Simon about how good he had been. 'But I'm sure you'll be just as good, Gary!' I reassured his successor.

Funding is based on my annual support plan which runs from April to March. Sometimes I don't fully spend. A lot of the training has halted in lockdown because of its practical nature. Catheter training is one example. Driver training is another. Defensive driving training involves ensuring that journeys are risk free and keeping me safe.

I have to itemise and justify all the different areas where spending is needed - training, PAs wages, courses, consumables and advertising. The clinical commission assess it and sign off the amount they think you need. The figures are audited every year.

Manual handling training is the worst. It gets a bit annoying being rolled on the bed ten times or so. Sometimes I wish someone else could be the dummy. COVID has limited it to four at a time, three plus the trainer, Beth. She is really nice and knows me well. She is a physio and does work for Cherry Training, a company set up by my friend Anne-Marie Mason and her husband David. Among other things they provide disabled people with access to enriching training opportunities. I use them for all my training. Anne-Marie has been a huge part of my life post-Alder Hey and the two of them have provided lots of training for my PAs. I can talk things through with Beth beforehand if I have concerns. That's really helpful and kind. In July 2021 I told her I was stressed as I didn't have anything else to focus on. She understood and said that I needed to get back to work.

Getting COVID tests for the PAs was obviously a key issue. Dad managed to sort it which he was pleased about. He started to administer them in January 2021, turning them round in half an hour. We had vaccine appointments offered at the end of January 2021. I had to fill forms online for each of my team, nine times over, which took a while. I couldn't force them which could be tricky but they had all had them by mid-

February. In the end they had been able to book their own. It became available as they were health and social care persons. The rules changed after I'd done all the form filling! All my PAs are very sensible and didn't want to put anyone at risk through lockdown. If they were unwell in any way they wouldn't come in. We've been very fortunate in that regard.

I had my first COVID jab on 3rd February, having got a message at short notice. I had to report to Kingsmead Medical Centre for thirteen minutes past four and I was home by five. I was a bit anxious about it all, I don't really know why. I suppose it was just typical of me. Maybe the fact that I had not being out for a while preyed on my mind or possibly which vaccine I was going to have. It was really well-organised. I was in and out in a flash. I had the Astra Zeneca one in the end. I felt a bit hot at night but that was not unusual for me. Then I couldn't sleep a wink. On the following night I just wasn't good. I had a temperature and my chest was rattling, as well as me being over-tired from the night before. I got worked up and teary. I rang Mum and Dad at about half past eleven. They asked if I wanted them to come over but I told them not to. I went to my room and got really upset then calmed myself down, sending Mum and Dad a text saying not to worry, that I'd be fine - and I was. Barbara and Gala were really good with me because I can be a bit of a nightmare in those situations. Gala always seems to say the right things at times like this. I was lying on my bed once in 2021 feeling awful and suggesting that I didn't want to be alive any more. Mum was really finding it hard and Gala said, 'What, just because you've got shits!?' Both were really brilliant at that point.

I spoke to Sarah on the next night and she said that Dan, her brother, hadn't been feeling well and he had had the jab around the same time as I. Naomi had had a sore throat. SHARKK WhatsApped me to say how excited they were for me. 'So pleased for you.' Susan added that she was five months pregnant with a girl. Lovely news! I also had my second jab in Kingsmead. Again, I was straight in and out. I treated myself to a trip into the nearby Tesco Express for some tangerines. I had a reaction (to the injection, not the tangerines!) and my temperature rose to 39 degrees.

The application process for new PAs is similar to the way it always has been. I normally advertise on Gumtree, Indeed or the Job Centre. I used the local newspaper for a while but no one looks there anymore and it was expensive. If anyone shows an interest in a position within the team I send them a job description and an application form. I ask for an email to ensure receipt. Quite often I don't get a reply for ages possibly because the job description sounds so scary. More recently we have had to accommodate the needs of the pandemic with interviews on Zoom. The first such interview went really well but it was weird. We had the mute/unmute issue that has become so common in online meetings. We couldn't hear the candidate. Mum sat next to me saying that we should have got Dad to do this. 'Have faith,' I said. Janet is certainly pleased that, with time being restricted on Zoom meetings, she doesn't have to listen to me droning on and on for quite so long in interviews!

It has become normal for me to interview with Mum and Janet and we have taken an increasingly informal approach over the years. I want to make people feel comfortable. The down side of doing it online is that interviewees cannot come to see me 'live', so to speak. Ideally, candidates need to know what kind of environment they might be entering by visiting my home. We had to accept, though, that certain normal parts of the process couldn't take place in lockdown.

What is most important is getting on with me and embracing the job. We start with a shadow shift, followed by the manual handling course.

Occasionally, there are setbacks with unexpected circumstances leading to PAs and candidates having to depart or withdraw but over the twenty years I've been so fortunate to have kept a stable core of dedicated staff. I know that any of them would help me at the drop of a hat if I rang needing something. They have been so supportive. I must have burst into tears on all of them at some point or other! It is important to have coping strategies when situations turn pear-shaped. I had a situation where a PA resigned after just joining. Dealing with adversity like that is all part of life's learning process.

I have been doing appraisals for some years now. They have developed into a recognisable pattern. We do them quarterly, trying to fit in with duty periods. Mum minutes them. I want to know how people are and what improvements can be made. They are also opportunities to thank my staff for all they do. I know that I need to learn to talk more slowly and avoid interrupting people. The chats are supposed to be 20% me talking, 80% them. I'm nowhere near those figures! Having verbal diarrhoeia doesn't help! Mind you, most of my friends are as bad!

I worry before I have full meetings with all my team. Usually Mum will be with me but in March 2021 I hosted one on my own. I was so nervous but it went well. It was about forty-five minutes long. It was fine. I didn't need to have worried. How many times have I said that to myself?!

It is always nice to get together outside the work environment and, sadly, these opportunities have been few and far between recently. At the end of February 2020, we all went to the Hollies for a burger. It was a special offer. I had been with work a couple of times and took the PAs on the strength of it. Then lockdown came. We had lunch outside at a pub in October 2020 but I can't wait for the next time. A strong bond can develop over time. Heated situations are few and far between. Simon came from Southport once and said,

'Hannah, I don't know how you have such a settled team. A lot of the people I deal with have staff who come and go so much quicker and don't have the training in place as well as you do.'

That made me feel so proud.

The PA has a stock of regular recognisable tasks to do each shift. Regular requirements include getting me washed, up and into my chair, sorting out my bladder and my bowels, applying medication at regular intervals throughout the day, making my lunch and tea and attending to specific needs like my laptop. I have two people in the morning between nine and one. There's a lot of manual handling in that period. It takes two to get me up and dressed. One might wash my hair while the other walks Mabel.

That's the predictable course of events but with me being me you never know what unexpected treats might happen...! I think back over the years to television and radio interviews, trips to the shops and holidays. The life of a PA is never dull!

We have been changing the pay roll details and I spoke to Janet to get her to sort it. It's such a relief when I can delegate stuff. Janet said at one point, 'Remember when you were first lumbered with me.' I'm saying to her, 'Janet, you don't know how much you help me and what you've done for me.' When Janet had COVID I really missed her and had to do her work with Mum.

Managing a team requires strength and a lot of responsibility. That is not something that always rests easily with me. The PAs often appreciate what I do and make kind comments but sometimes I think that I try too hard to want people to like me and, consequently, my head gets mashed up. I worry that they don't like the way I do things, even though I know that it is what they have signed up for. My sisters tell me that every one of them has a choice about whether they are here or not.

I can still have stressful days over seemingly small issues. In my effort to try to please people all the time things like time sheets can bother me although the last year has taught me that these are the things that don't matter as much. I even worried about paying my PAs too early before Christmas 2020 when Janet wasn't available to help Mum and I.

I am definitely guilty of overthinking things and blowing situations up out of all proportions. I must learn to control my paranoia. Jess and Naomi tell me that I worry when I have nothing to worry about. I'm worrying more about the people who work here than my own family. My face will go bright red and I can feel my heart beating fast. One night I totally flipped my lid with one of the PAs. After I had lost it, I rang Mum. She let me swear like a trooper. I sounded such a horrible person but

Mum reassured me that I wasn't that sort of person naturally and not to change who I was. Things returned to normal but it made me think that perhaps that is a better way of dealing with situations than stewing over things for ages. In that respect I wish I was more like Jess because she is able to deal with issues that way. I find that I can be honest, direct and critical to my family but it's different with my carers.

It's lovely when my carers show empathy towards me. I was chatting with Nichola one day and told her she needed to be patient with me.

'You kidding?' she replied. 'You are the most patient person I've ever met. You are amazing.'

She went on to ask me what I missed the most in my situation.

'Being on my own, doing my own hair, getting in the shower. Mainly being on my own.'

Nichola showed empathy that day and I appreciated it. People can forget how hard my situation is.

I'd give anything to be on my own for just a day. I know that I have sacrificed the chance to be alone and it is difficult to bear at times. One day Helga and Gala were swapping shifts and putting the bins out. They shut my front door behind them briefly because the cold was getting in. Mabel and I were ON OUR OWN!!! I was on Houseparty with Jess and Naomi and shouting, 'I'M ON MY OWN! YAY! I'M ON MY OWN IN THE HOUSE!'

They were telling me to say something controversial.

'I HATE EVERYONE!' was what I came up with.

I don't, of course, but just at that moment in time I felt like saying something mad...I was going really stupid but then Gala came back into the house and I had to shut up. For two minutes I had been by myself. It was the best thing ever!

At Mum and Dad's when they are moving the cars they will say, 'You'll be alright for a minute won't you?'

''YEAH. Absolutely! Can't you just go out for ten minutes and leave me and Mabel?'

'No!'

'Why not?' Nothing's going to happen.'
'How do you know that?'
'I just want to be on my own for a few minutes.'

The only other time that I'm on my own is if someone pops into a shop and leaves me in the car. I'll talk to myself and wonder what the people in the next car might be thinking. If Dad pops into ALDI and about fifty people come out who went in after him I'll be shouting, 'WHERE ARE YOU?' People who see me must think I'm crackers!

I can still have really bad days but then everyone does. Occasionally. I know my situation and can't change it. I don't have to like it. I still find it hard when I see others doing things that I will never do. I wish I could just jump into a front seat of a car and drive somewhere.

CHAPTER FIFTEEN

Friends for Life

I turned round immediately, put my wheelchair on speed three and poor old Barbara was having to jog back with me!

I hadn't been in my new house very long when Anna FaceTimed me with news of her engagement to Jim. It was really nice. We had been waiting for ages for an announcement because they had been going out since university days. She added jokingly that they were thinking of Hawaii for the service. I selfishly said, 'Don't. I'll not get there!' In the end they opted for their local church. It was July 2017 and all of SHARKK were there.

For the hen 'do' we had gone to Chester Races. I remember the day well because I was there before any of the others. Gala came with me and got dressed up for the occasion. There was a lot of fun and the weather was nice. There had been a get together in Delamere the night before at the Fish Pool restaurant. I had had a lovely catch up with friends I'd not seen for ages.

I enjoyed getting ready for the wedding. I opted to sit in the vestry, for a better view. I was so glad that I did because I got very emotional. I couldn't stop crying, so much so that I was gasping for breath at one point. I wore myself out with the effort. I can't really explain why I was overwhelmed other than to describe it as a mixture of emotions which is difficult to explain. Kate and Susan could see me from the front pew in the church and were mouthing, 'Are you alright?' Despite my troubles it was a lovely wedding. Lizzy and Sarah sang.

I've known Anna's family for years so it was good to see them. My friends tended to my every need at the reception, which was held in a local village near where I live. The room looked a picture and I stayed for ages. We danced the night away. Mum had been there for the wedding and hung around in the background because she wanted it to be for me and my friends. It is very rare for us to be all together but they are always with me in spirit.

Christmas 2019 was probably the first meet-up since Anna's wedding over two years earlier. We went to a local pub. A PA took me. We had our own area which was nice. Rosanne was pregnant, Anna and Kate had their babies there. How SHARKK meetings have changed over the years! We stayed for the whole evening.

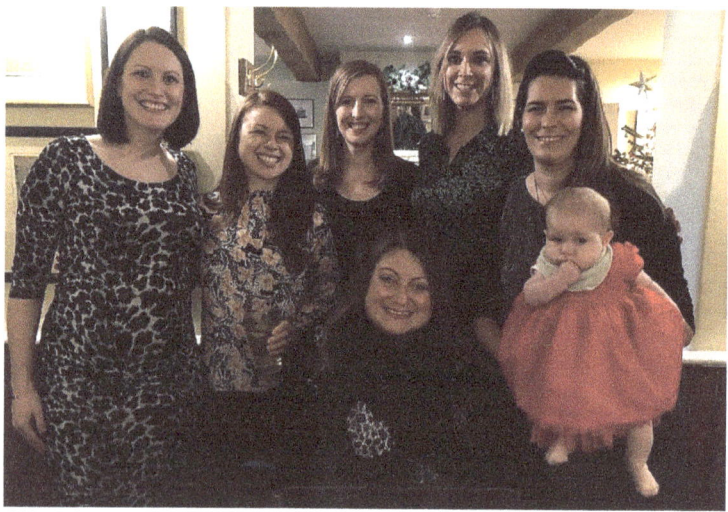

SHARKK plus one! (L to R, Rosanne, Kate, Susan, Karen & Anna with daughter Chloe)

Mum brought the book of pictures from the wedding in Italy when she came back later and showed it round. It was so nice for me to be featured on them for once. I had had my tattoo just several days before and showed it off. They thought it was brilliant! As I thought back in the early weeks of the new year, with the pandemic taking a grip, I was convinced that we would not meet again like that for some time, particularly with those living abroad who might not be able to fly for ages.

I feel so privileged and lucky to have kept the company and friendship of these unbelievable people. I wouldn't have done as much as I have if I hadn't pushed myself to try all the things that they were doing. Our paths since school have taken us far and wide but distance has never hindered the strength of our bond. Lockdown has certainly not stopped us communicating by various media but, occasionally, a surprise visit has done me the world of good.

I was walking Mabel near home with Barbara when I got a call from Anna. She was on my drive! I knew she was in Cheshire but not that close to me! When lockdown happened she was in Delamere with her mum and dad. I had only spoken to her a couple of days earlier, on the phone, and we agreed that we needed to get together. I didn't realise it would be this quick! I thought it would have to be a walk in Delamere Forest or something like that. For some reason I had decided to go down the local farm road instead of going into Northwich and I'm so glad I did. I turned round immediately, put my wheelchair on speed three and poor old Barbara was having to jog back with me! She told me that she didn't need the gym after that work out! As for Mabel, she had to run as well as she was attached to my chair!

It was worth it. I'd not seen Anna in 'real life' for a year. Then Mum rang and I told her what had happened. She said,

'Guess where I've been? Delamere Forest! I thought that I might have met Anna and Maureen (her Mum) in the forest but now I know she was at your house!'

We had to stay outside but Anna's visit really cheered me up. I was buzzing! She didn't have to do that at such a difficult time but it is typical of the spontaneity within my group.

My friends and I chat all the time. Through COVID we have talked even more. We discuss all the subjects under the sun. Someone had told Karen that she looked like a computer nerd on a picture from school and she thanked us all for sticking with her. Someone else said, 'I think we all did.' Then someone found a picture of Karen in leopard print. I said she'd lent me that at a disco in Austria... and on we went to the next subject!

In April 2021 I got another call from Anna, giving me some fresh news. I expected it to be that she was having another baby but it wasn't. She was moving back to Cheshire as Jim had got a job in Manchester. I knew it was on the cards but not this quickly. I was so happy,

'It's the best news I've ever had,' I exaggerated in typical Hannah fashion!

I rang Mum to tell her and was so excited that I just could not stop crying. Anna's news made me think again of the love of my friends and everything we have shared. It came at a good time as I had been dealing with some issues at home which had been bothering me. I think that I just needed a release and she had provided it.

Those first fifteen years are so precious and important to me. When I'm in with my friends we talk about High School a lot. They were very important days, meeting up and establishing some brilliant new friendships. On another occasion Karen WhatsApped all of SHARKK from Barcelona where she organises photo shoots. She had just bought a beautiful house on the harbour at Sitges. It was Grandma and Grandpa's favourite place for holidays. I really want to go there sometime because Grandpa always said how beautiful it was and I couldn't get to Karen's wedding there because we were going to France near that time. Karen told us that she had walked into the kitchen where she worked and they had Roberts Bread, made about two miles from my house!

I really enjoy seeing the children of my friends. Rosanne FaceTimed one day and I had a lengthy chat with her and eight-month-old Benjamin who kept putting things in the washing machine and taking them out again. This must have amused him for about twenty minutes! Rosanne lives in St Albans so her mum and dad have seen little of little Benjamin during the pandemic.

For a birthday treat I went to Davenports Tea Rooms a few miles from home with Lizzy, Sarah and Lizzy's twins, Lottie and Ellie. Davenports is 'olde worlde' and there is an Alice in Wonderland feel.

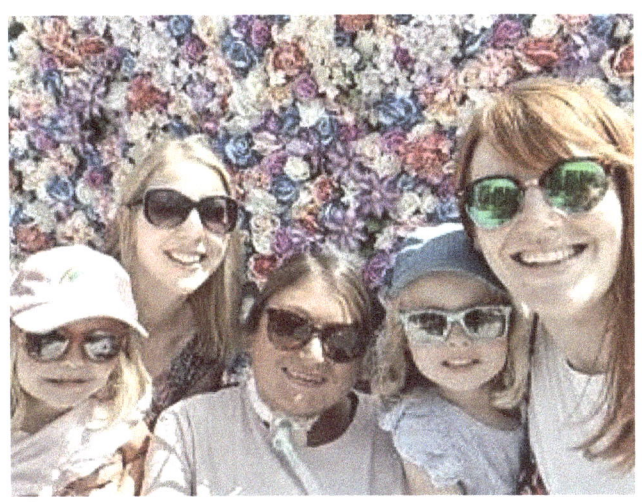

I was so impressed with the Tea Rooms that I got them to send me an afternoon tea on 20th May. That's the day when I always do something different because it is the day when I first went into hospital. With lockdown I was limited so I arranged a surprise tea for Mum and Dad. I had planned it a few days before. I remembered that I didn't have a nice table cloth so ordered one from Amazon. I then realised that I didn't have a cake stand. The PAs had bought me one when I moved in but it was at Mum and Dad's house. I couldn't risk letting them into my secret so asked my PAs if anyone had one. We sorted it.

    I chose a Friday because Dad didn't work that day. I dressed up and got the conservatory looking nice with bunting. I rang Mum and Dad and asked if they had plans for the day. Could they come round about one o'clock? They thought that Dad had a conference call then. 'Oh no!' I thought to myself. They came later in the afternoon and I asked them to open the box. It had been decorated very nicely. They were so pleased and we had a lovely afternoon. It's rare that I can keep something a surprise so I was proud of myself.

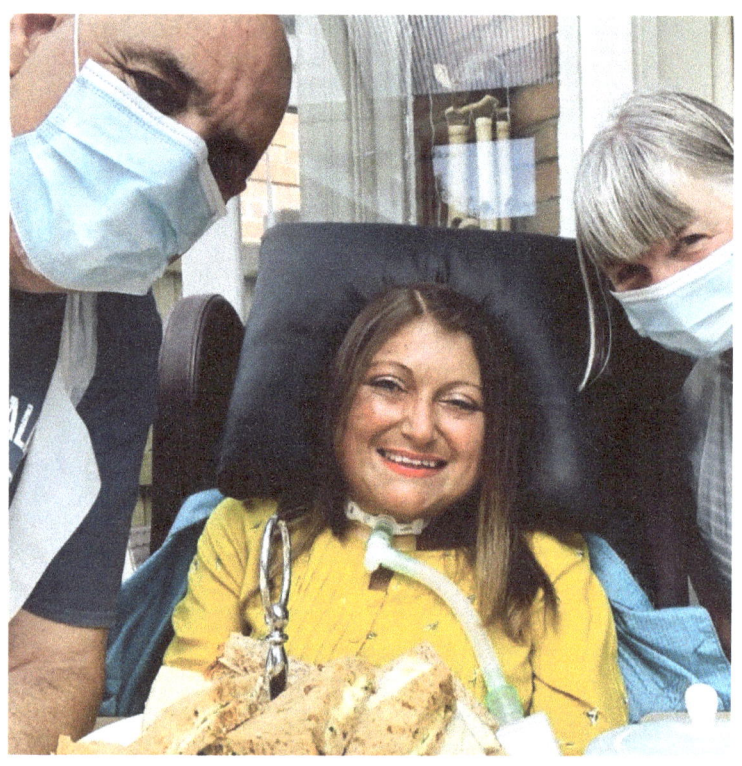

Celia is a special friend despite not being one of our year group. She is Susan's younger sister and you may remember me mentioning her in previous books. I was sending her WhatsApps while I was on the computer and she said, 'Oh my God, Hannah, remember when you couldn't do any of that sort of thing?' I remember Celia being concerned about how many emails I had in my Inbox. I updated her on the figure and she almost had a heart attack! 23500, or something. I can't be bothered to face them all, they are all rubbish. I need to unsubscribe to so many things. It's going to be a million one day!

    Celia does not get back home often so it was lovely to share a walk with her around the beginning of March 2021. It was her birthday the day before mine. I met her at Witton Mill just behind Northwich Tip. Her dad, Stephen, dropped her off and it was lovely to see him as well. Mum was on the walk but stayed behind at a distance, meeting up with Stephen at one point. Celia and I had a lovely chat and catch up, probably the first time since last summer when we could go into each other's gardens. We took photos and watched Mabel get really wet running into water.

Celia has been doing a Hundred Happy Days on Facebook. Every day you submit a picture of something that makes you happy. It is making her realise how important it is to focus on good things. She is one of my closest friends. I know she will never judge me, whatever I tell her. She's been promoted at work and is doing extremely well. She's in the office at eight and I'm not even up until the afternoon!

Despite all the support and love within our group it would be taken to a whole new level of intensity when my spirits plummeted yet again towards the end of the summer 2021. More about that later.

CHAPTER SIXTEEN

My Lovely Bunch of Roses

'I started to get very emotional and cried for an hour'

My fabulous family continue to be at the heart of my world and my love for them has been ever more obvious during recent months when circumstances have conspired to keep them at bay for days at a time.

I've always been in close touch with my sisters, Jess and Naomi, but probably even more so during the pandemic. We have talked for hours about the most random things and are always having a go at each other! For my twentieth anniversary of coming out of hospital Naomi and Jess bought me a cake. I told them that I might have preferred a Colin the Caterpillar cake. Jess's reply was unprintable but it made me laugh. I know she didn't mean it but I like the way we have banter like that. It's so refreshing to behave that way. On another occasion I was watching 'I'm a Celebrity' when one of the contestants was sick. Straight away my phone rang and it was Naomi. She knew I hated sick and wanted to warn me about it thinking I might be behind on the action, which I often am because I record a lot of programmes and pause the television frequently. On this occasion I was actually watching live and saw it at the same time! Not a pretty sight! My family have such a weird sense of humour and it really sparks me the way we don't pussy foot around each other. Toilet humour is still a favourite subject. We don't really grow up.

My mind is often back in the past enjoying family times. I spend a lot of time thinking back to our childhood. Visits to Marbury Park or Delamere Forest take me straight back to the eighties and nineties. I was saying to one of my PAs only the other day how much I enjoyed primary school. Mine was a lovely year group and it's nice that both Helen Mitchell and Edward Belcher from my class have moved back into Cheshire. Everything was so much fun back then. When we played schools I had to be the teacher because I was bossy. I remember Helen's birthday parties, putting pegs on a washing line and sucking peas up on a straw. That's one game that I can still do!

Childhood memories are precious to me. They are still so clear in my mind. Toast and jam at the Mitchells house. And mince. I always remember asking Dad if we could just have ordinary mince rather than something covered in fancy cooking ingredients. I still talk to my PAs about that. I often tell them stories from back then such as when I was in Northwich Infirmary with my sisters and the Mitchells while Gillian Mitchell was having stitches having fallen off a bench. An old lady was impressed with the patient way we were waiting and offered us sweets. I wouldn't let her because we weren't allowed to take sweets from strangers. The others weren't pleased with me! I remember watching the Miss World contest on a sleepover at our house. We were up late and screaming. Helen kicked the lamp over by accident. We had bagels. Mum always bought them up when she saw them in Sainsburys. Helen told me that the first thing she remembers having at our house was a bagel. She had never had one before and still to this day will think about the Roses when she eats one.

Weekends have always been special times for my family. The pandemic has inevitably restricted meeting up but on Sundays Dad always cooks and there is often food left over. One week in January 2021 I had enough vegetable stew for four successive nights! He made a Beef Wellington for the first time and it was gorgeous! One of the best things he's ever made. It was perfect. The best thing I've had in my life! Here I go again! Dave told me that I've used 'best' forty times in this book! I remember Dad making me some proper Jewish soup, something I'd been on about for ages.

'Why don't you do it?' I had kept asking him.

'Well, I had it every week growing up, that's why.'

Anyway, he finally relented and it was delicious. Dumplings, noodles, the lot.

On some Sundays I get a bit emotional going back to the family home as I remember all the special big family get togethers at weekends with grandparents and lovely meals which, hopefully, will return on a regular basis.

There's nothing better than holiday time with the five Roses but I also love trips with some of the famous five. I remember Mum taking me to Crufts in 2019. That sounds as if she was exhibiting me! Mum drove us and it was the first time that I stayed long enough to watch a Best in Breed section. I'd always wanted to see the Gundogs section and that's what happened. I didn't have to think about rushing back. I was looking on when I got a message from Nicola at work. She was watching the programme, spotted me and sent some pictures of me on television! I had a massive Subway cup in front of my face looking really bored! That was an unfortunate image because I had had a really good day. Mum less so. At one point she said that if I watched much more I would get a deep-vein thrombosis! Ha! Ha! I was really excited that the Labrador won and as I was walking out of the arena I met the winning owner with her dog! I asked her for a picture, of course! Celebrity hunter! She was from Macclesfield, only about twenty miles from me. I told her about Mabel who wasn't with us on that occasion. It would have got her too excited!

Lockdown played havoc with many wedding celebrations, including Naomi's. I felt so sorry for her and Dan. Luckily they were both chilled about it and have that incredible mentality that they know there's nothing that they can do about the situation. Grandpa had been a jeweller and kept some wedding rings back. Naomi and Dan were able to choose from them and, at last, they got married in June 2021. It was a lovely family occasion despite the restrictions that still applied.

We were allowed thirty people and Naomi had two friends. Jess and I were bridesmaids along with Naomi's friend Lisa. Ahead of the day I did a trial run to the venue in Liverpool, which was helpful. With limited space in the lift I knew that I would need my manual wheelchair.

As previously mentioned, we organised Naomi's hen party online and then held it in Mum and Dad's garden with COVID safe games and afternoon tea. Mum made scones; Dad made cakes. It was not what we have become accustomed to these days for hen parties but the restrictions placed on us enabled us to organise something different and we all enjoyed the occasion in beautiful weather. Loads of Naomi's friends from school and Liverpool were there. We played a game where we each said a truth and a lie about her. Here's mine,

'She once tipped someone out of a wheelchair.

She once met the band Blue.'

I think the answer's pretty obvious!

Jess wore a straw hat which I said made her look like Peggy Patch. She maintained she didn't know who I was talking about. I explained that she was on the children's programme 'Playdays'. 'The Mitchells had a Peggy Patch' I told her. In bed that night I found a picture of Peggy on Google and sent it to our WhatsApp group. I did it three times by accident but I did it.

Barbara came into work on the day of the wedding, specially to do my dressings so that Mum didn't have to get me ready. Michaela and her took me to Liverpool. I had to be there by noon for a three o'clock start. Mum and Dad met us outside and I was soon with Naomi and the bridesmaids having hair and make-up done.

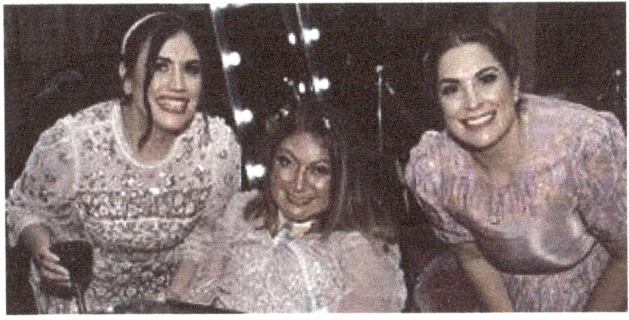

The photographer was also a hypnotherapist and probably regretted telling us that after fielding dozens of questions from us for about an hour! It was a lovely chilled atmosphere.

We all got teary when we saw Naomi in her dress. It was the hotel's first wedding for ages so we didn't know what the procedure was for going down the aisle. I went in first, pushed by Mum. The room was laid out really nice. There was plenty of space. Dan looked nervous, typical of a groom. It was a sweet and lovely service.

No one in the congregation knew what to answer for, 'Would you look after Dan and Naomi'. The celebrant was not impressed by our mumbled and mixed answers so we repeated it again. 'WE WILL!' came back strongly from across the room, raising a smile! We went up to the roof of the hotel for drinks and canapés with family we hadn't seen for ages. There was a lovely intimacy about it.

Dad's speech was really good and included how Dan had asked him for permission to marry his youngest daughter. We heard about Naomi trapping her fingers under a toilet seat and getting her legs stuck through railings at the White House. Someone looking like Sylvester Stallone had run across the road with a crowbar. Dad described the day when Naomi left a note for the tooth fairy, demanding £5. Naomi told him not to talk about when she was cruel to the pets. Her plea made no difference. He told us! It was a familiar wedding speech by a father stitching up his daughter with embarrassing memories!

Dan's speech was so lovely. I started to get very emotional and cried for an hour, as did Jess. She gets upset when I am and vice versa. It was a mixture of emotions for me. Jess helped me with a perpetually runny nose which eventually bled. She sent Stuart out to get some tissues. I cried through the best man's speech. He told how Dan proposed outside the toilet door in the hotel room in Paris. We heard his chat up line on first meeting Naomi in Liverpool's Bumpers Night Club. 'How old are you?'

It was lovely to catch up with our cousins and get to know Dan's side of the family. At the end of the day, I was picked up at about half past ten tired and emotional, which continued through the following day. I'd got through well. There was just a short period when I had felt faint and unwell but I powered through.

We had a separate get together some time after the wedding, once COVID restrictions had been eased. This was an opportunity to invite friends and family who might not have been able to attend the wedding service. I was really looking forward to catching up with everybody. It was at Blakemere Village, just a mile or two up Chester Road. My friend Vicky did my make-up for the day and we arrived together. That was so nice of her. We had such a good time and I really appreciated her being there with me. I love this picture of the two of us.

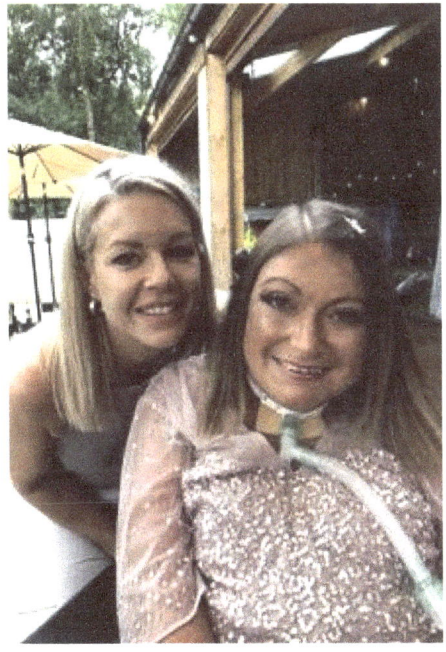

There was plenty for guests to see and do, including a Falconry display. At one point the guy asked Naomi and Dan to kiss and as they did one of the large birds flew in between them! It was exciting to feel one brush my hair as it flew past me. Anna, Jim and Chloe had only just moved back north and it was lovely that they could be there. Sue fell off the Segway which it is impossible to fall off! Little Hughie now thinks every party will be like that in future! He's going to be disappointed.

Between the wedding and the party Naomi and Dan bought a puppy. They had said they might when they were married but I wasn't sure that Dan was that keen. Naomi sent me a message to say they were going to see a litter of puppies that belonged to Dan's friend's Mum. They are like labradors crossed with a sheepdog. I was urging Naomi to get one, preferably a girl for company for Mabel, but she insisted that they were going to be sensible and take their time. Next thing I know she's sending me a picture of Dan holding a puppy with the caption, 'Meet Betty Buckney'!!! I think that I was more excited than them as I video called. It wasn't long before I was heading across to Liverpool to meet the new addition. It was the first time I'd visited Naomi's house and it was to see her puppy! It was so accessible and I got straight through to the back garden to meet the tiny, shy Betty. Mabel was the first dog that she had met and they were so lovely together, licking each other's faces. I think that Mabel started to mother her. It was the beginning of a lovely friendship.

I really looked forward to celebrating Mum's birthday in 2021. I was going round and having a take away with her and Dad. Naomi had arranged to be at the door with presents, not being able to come in because of COVID restrictions. Unfortunately, Jess was at work. I bought Mum a scarf. I thought it was so nice that I bought one for myself! I also got her a bouquet of Turkish Delight, looking like flowers.

2021 was a milestone year for Dad. He was 70 years old, celebrated retirement and a Ruby anniversary with Mum. We all wanted to do something really special for his birthday. Naomi, Jess and I worked together to get a signed Sergio Aguero shirt, even though he was no longer at Manchester City. We looked everywhere. Some cost as much as £700! Jess kept hold of it until we took it to the Panoramic in Liverpool for our birthday meal on the Sunday before his birthday the next day. It was a five-course tasting menu and gorgeous. We presented him with the framed shirt at the table. He was very excited.

I had decided to put together a book of pictures from his life and there were many occasions when I wish that I hadn't! Using only my mouth to edit, the book took me for ever! I nearly gave up after the first page! It was really hard keeping it a secret from Dad. Then I discovered that it wasn't going to come on time so I had to redo it in a different style with more pictures required. It still didn't arrive on time. I was so mad because I'd put so much effort into it and even paid extra for a delivery on the day. I also got Grandma Frances and Aunty Ellen mixed up. Despite all that, Dad was so touched.

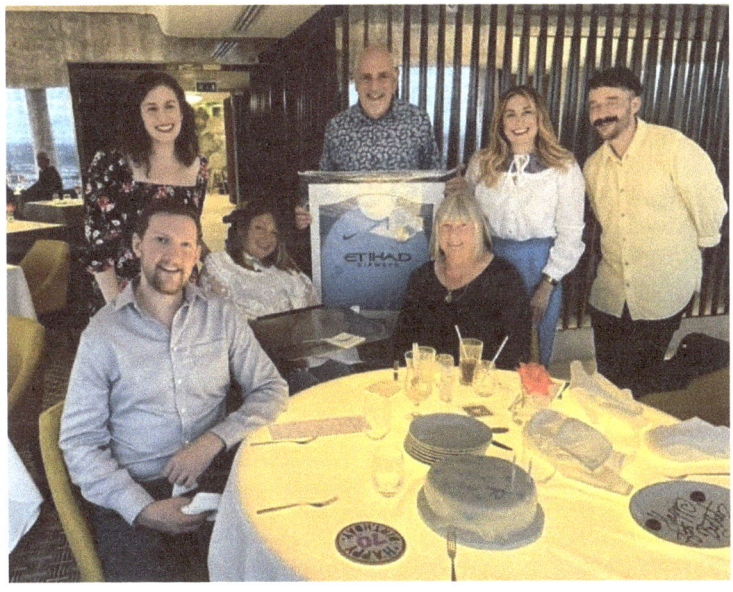

Mum's 70th birthday followed a few months later and I wanted to prepare a book of pictures similar to Dad's. It took for ever because Dad had to find all the pictures and we shared dozens and dozens of WhatsApp messages clarifying when the pictures were taken. I also arranged for a series of video messages from her relatives in Ireland. Jess's friend, Candy, kindly put the presentation together for me and told us, 'I've never heard anyone sound so Irish in all my life!' Mum watched it on her birthday and loved it!

I was so happy that Dad was retiring but it was not the best start. He had to look after Mum who had gone down with COVID, I was not feeling great and Naomi's puppy was staying at theirs!

I still think a lot about my grandparents. In a way I'm so glad that they haven't been around through COVID. It's so hard to imagine just thinking of grandpa, Dad's father, in a house on his own. I remember that Dad always rang grandpa on his way home from work. With Mum's mother, Grandma Frances, being in the care home it would have been horrific. She just wanted someone to be in there every day and we wouldn't have been able to do that with the heavy restrictions imposed. I have so many happy memories of my grandparents and when I'm not regaling the PAs with stories from my childhood I'm talking about them, particularly around birthdays or anniversaries of their deaths.

We were talking about cats one day and Mum was in on the conversation. She recalled working in a car showroom, Lookers, as a receptionist and a man came in and said that he had a set of kittens which he was going to get rid of as he didn't want them anymore. Mum immediately took one and hid it in the shed at home, giving it food and water. Grandma Frances found out and let her have it in the house until the kitten knocked over a vase of flowers and the water ran down into the television, making it useless. Grandma Frances didn't see animals as pets. She grew up on a farm with cats and dogs but they were working animals. She really liked Bella and Mabel, though. We laughed about the time when Bella ate the heel off her shoe. We recalled how Grandma always used to say. 'Oh Jesus, Mary and Joseph!' in her engaging Irish lilt.

I can't complete book three without giving Nicky a mention. He is Dad's cousin and was really close to grandpa. He has three children and we see a lot of him and his family. I always refer to him as 'Dad's cousin' instead of by his name and this has become a source of humour over the years! Nicky will often say, 'I'm your dad's cousin!' to me. We have talked about him not getting a mention yet in the books so here's a special call out for 'Dad's cousin'!

One very special part of our family passed away at the end of 2020. Adele Rose was an inspiration to me. When I mention her name I guarantee that many of you will immediately wonder where you've heard that before. The answer is on Coronation Street. Adele was not only the first female writer on the Street but she has also written more episodes than any other writer on the programme. She wrote 457 scripts over a period of thirty-seven years from 1961.

Grandad's brother Monty was married to Adele. Monty was a Manchester doctor. One of the American cousins saw my Facebook profile picture and told me I looked like him. Dad got a picture of him and it was true. I messaged my family,

'Hey, you can't say I've got an Irish face anymore because I've been told I look like a Jewish man.'

This strong, successful lady was a big influence on me so her death came as a shock. Her daughter Carrie had passed away from sepsis around the time when I moved in to my new house. In Adele's case it was pneumonia. Dad spoke to her son Stephen a few times. Stephen could imagine the two of them up there drinking champagne! There have been some lovely pieces written about her and Ant and Dec tweeted a tribute connected with 'Byker Grove', the show which started their careers,

'We are very sad to hear of the passing of Adele Rose, the creator of Byker Grove. She was an incredible lady and a wonderful writer. We will always be grateful for what she did for us and the north east. Thank you, Adele, and rest in peace.'

Adele specialised in developing strong female characters, none more so than Elsie Tanner off 'Coronation Street'. I didn't realise until after her death that she had been the bridesmaid of Pat Phoenix (who played Elsie) when she remarried! Writer Jack Rosenthal encouraged her in her writing and it is a nice twist that his wife Maureen Lipman is playing Evelyn Plummer, yet another strong female character, on Corrie at the moment.

You might remember that I did a degree in Media and Crime. I asked Adele for information on writing a soap and found what she had sent only quite recently! It was really interesting to read it all back. Apparently, one character always used to complain about the lines she had written (and that was Julie Goodyear).

Adele gets a mention in the following typically random snippet of conversation between myself and my friend Joanne,

Hannah	Adele passed away
Joanne	Are you going to the funeral?
Hannah	Probably not because it was yesterday
Joanne	Well you won't if it was yesterday, will you!

I'm sure that Adele would have had a smile at that and maybe even fitted it into a Corrie script!

CHAPTER SEVENTEEN

Joanne

'Whoever says, "I missed you coming?!" to the gas man!?'

Since my second book was published I have gained a new friend who is really rather special. I have already mentioned her in passing but I want to give her a proper mention in this book. Joanne and I met through the Back Up scheme when I acted as her mentor. It was March 2020 but it seems a lot further back than that. The idea was to arrange a number of calls, about ten, at a mutually convenient time. We found that we clicked immediately. We were about the same age, had a similar sense of humour and common interests. I asked Back Up if I could continue my contact with her beyond the statutory period. They were really pleased to agree. I'm glad that they did because Joanne has brought a new perspective into my life. What has happened to me is like a quarter of the issues that she has had to deal with. Sadly, she is unable to see the world around her like I can but despite all her problems she is assertive and positive.

Our relationship has blossomed. Talking to Joanne has helped me enormously and been a bonus through lockdown. Absolutely nothing is private between us. Our chats are frequently long, usually random and covering a huge range of subjects. One day we discussed how hard it was not having our own personal space and having to say to PAs, 'Can you shut the door?' On another we spent an hour talking about 'Saved by the Bell', the American sitcom.

There has always been something fresh to talk about with Joanne. We never dry up. She texted me once about a dream that she had had whilst lying in bed,

'I was on 'Steph's Packed Lunch' on Channel 4. I was telling Steph about when you and I had first met and I was getting quite emotional. It was just after that conversation we had had on Friday about how hard it is with carers and stuff. Then Steph started crying as did everyone. Steph said "Jo, we have a surprise for you" and you appeared on Zoom. It wasn't good enough for me but then you came in in real life and we got to hug for the first time.'

She told me mid-chat one day that she'd gone to school with Tom from McFly!

'Wow! Why didn't you tell me that?' I asked her.

'Well, you never told me that your dad was Father Christmas,' was her reply.

We chatted once about how frustrating Siri is for people who can't type. She had asked for my address. Davenham became David M then Dagenham. One time I was on with her when the gas man arrived. He had been delayed by COVID so I needed to see him. He sorted things out for me. He was really nice and it was such a change to see a friendly face interacting with me. Joanne heard me talking to him in the background,

'Oh my God, Hannah, are you flirting?! No one flirts with their gas man!' Whoever says, "I missed you coming?!" to the gas man!?'

Maybe one day a service man will arrive and we'll just get married.

Inevitably, we share common frustrations. One is when someone is helping you to complete a task but telling a story at the same time. We both agreed that our mums are the worst at this. Yes, it's nice to be sociable but inside you are just urging them to get on with the dressings or getting you dressed and there they are having a chat as if tomorrow will do! Now I start putting the Benny Hill theme music on when Mum's there. She gets the point and quickens up immediately. Yes, I want a sociable Mum but there's a time and a place.

It's also frustrating when one of us is poorly, then the other and contact becomes less regular between us. We both share frustrations about people we have organised to do something then not turning up. This is a topic that I've previously covered in my books. People don't always understand the effort that has gone in to getting ourselves ready for an appointment or visit.

We have discussed doing a podcast. Hopefully it will happen one day. Podcasts are so popular at the moment and ours will be called 'Spinal Chat', a name which came from Naomi. We decided that we should let the world hear some of our crazy chats. In the initial stages, I got a lot of help from Sam Fielding, a friend of Dave's. They worked together at Fleetwood Town Football Club. Sam was so helpful and made me feel that I could do the podcast production myself.

I told my friends on a WhatsApp chat about the idea. They thought it was just amazing! They were so excited for me and we spoke about having guests on, like themselves. Despite all they have done for me they couldn't believe why I might consider them.

It was through practising for the podcast that I saw Joanne for the first time. We had arranged a practice but I was beginning to have second thoughts as I'd had my flu jab the day before and not got much sleep overnight. Mum had told me to have a quieter day but when she turned up I was getting ready to go out with Mabel. Then I got a message from Joanne asking if I could put it back half an hour which helped. There were a few hurdles to get over before we started.

For the first ten minutes I was just sitting waiting for her to come on. She sent me a text to say, 'Bear with me'. Then, suddenly, I could see her ceiling! Moments later, I saw her! It was the first time that I had actually seen Joanne in her room.

'Can you hear me?'
'Yes!'

It was so weird after we had been chatting for so long. I looked like a robot with my possum and microphone in front of me. One ear phone into the computer, one into my phone. We spoke for about an hour, taking the micky out of each other as always. I had a mini-crisis at the end when I thought that I hadn't recorded it! How would I tell Joanne after she had done so well? All was fine in the end. I couldn't believe the two of us had achieved it what with both our sets of issues. Neither of us had any help. Dad was well-impressed.

'Hopefully, we will end up really famous and rich and able to buy a house in Spain!' said Joanne.

'Oh my God, that message really made me cry,' I replied. 'I hope this is you looking into the future and what you see is going to happen.'

Jess's husband Stuart has done a jingle for me. I need to think of topics for each show as well as having the chatty element. It must stay natural. It'll happen one day and one day Joanne and I will meet. I'm sure of that.

CHAPTER EIGHTEEN

The Joys of Online Shopping

'One of the weirdest purchases had to be the jump suit.'

Those of you who know me well will be aware that I've always been fond of shopping, both out and about and online. During lockdown my interest online has turned into an obsession. Amazon Prime is just the best thing ever. I can fairly be described as participating to excessively crazy levels. Take this example, for instance. I really wanted to try a pickled egg one day so looked on Amazon and bought a jar. When it arrived, I tucked into my first and it was horrible! Six pounds wasted! I decided to pretend that they were a present, give them to Dad and hope that he wouldn't realise that one was missing. Dad made some of his own. I think he was trying to prove a point after I'd challenged him to make some. They were really nice if not as pickly as I would have wanted.

I've found some great deli places online with delights such as black pudding with chilli in, pork pies with black pudding in, truffle cheese and truffle crisps, caramelised nuts and spicy sausage. There's an Italian deli which has the same soft biscuits that we had in Italy and I've ordered some of them. You have to spend a certain amount, £30, to get the delivery. Sometimes, I don't know what I'm doing. I'm losing my mind trying to find the weirdest thing that I can have delivered to my house! One time I really wanted some seaweed that you can eat. It's healthy. They didn't have it on my ASDA shop so I tried Amazon.

'Dad?'

'What do you want now?'

'I can buy eighteen packs of seaweed for £9. I just want your advice. Is this good value?'

'Buy it if that's what you want. I can't believe you've rung me just to ask that question.'

That's just an example of how bored I have got during lockdown.

I ordered a cuddly sloth for Mabel. We suspected that there were mice in the garage and I ordered traps. There was a bottle of Malibu which I bought as a Secret Santa for one of my PAs. Then there was a jar of olives. One of the weirdest purchases had to be the jump suit. I've always wanted to get into one. It was hilarious and far from straightforward. Barbara and Sharon got it on me but trying to get it off with Karen and Michaela took even longer!

Amazon has become the go to answer far too frequently. 'We need a new smoke alarm.' Get it on Amazon. 'We need a new bulb for the bathroom.' Get it on Amazon. If the PAs complain that we've run out of pens I'll sort a new batch straight away with Amazon. A box of black pens arrived one day and it was so exciting!

I've made the mistake of ordering certain items by accident from my personal care budget. I've repaid, of course. I can't really maintain they are for a carer. A bottle of Malibu in the budget plan?! I don't think so!

As a result of all this activity, there must be an Amazon delivery every day to my house, sometimes twice! We're getting quite friendly with the Hermes man. 'Here's another one for her,' he will say as the PA on duty answers the door. I have become very good at ordering presents for my friends during lockdown. I got a really good cushion with Sarah's dog name on but, typically, I had to order one for myself as well! You can imagine how much cardboard builds up. Gala gets very excited about ripping the cardboard up for the bin, sometimes as early as half past seven in the morning.

Perhaps the most unusual online purchases among many strange ones have been the fish. Yes, you can have fish delivered off the van to your doorstep. I have used a firm called 'Aquatics to Your Door', following a dramatic period in my fish keeping career. I do love my fish tank and have become something of a fish geek having kept various types for years, way before I left Mum and Dad's house. Fish are such therapeutic creatures. I'll sometimes sit in front of the tank rather than the television! When I'm online with my sisters I will often excitedly show them the fish swimming around. The little dwarf aquatic frogs are such an entertainment. Jess and Naomi don't share my enthusiasm, sadly. 'Oh yeah, right...' is a typical reaction. It's a bit like me with Jess's cats.

I got refused fish once, at Pets at Home. I told them how many I had already and they said I shouldn't have any more in a tank that size. I'm a big customer at the garden centre in Winnington near Northwich. I know the staff well there and always get a warm welcome. Dad has even visited without me, showing me the tanks on FaceTime and trying to establish which kind of fish I want that way.

In January 2021 the tank was empty. I had got an African Albino Clawed Toad. It looked like a raw chicken according to my sisters but I was tempted and bought one a couple of years ago from Winnington. Well, it got bigger and bigger as it systematically ate everything in my tank! There were videos of other such toads online. One man said that you could even feed them Kentucky Fried Chicken!

I had turned into a fish killer! It got to the stage where I didn't want it in my tank any more. Every time Janet came to do the timesheets I had to put a cover over the tank – it was so disgusting and distracting. I knew that it couldn't just be thrown away or flushed down the toilet. One of the carers suggested it be thrown into the river but Dad was concerned about it mutating and throwing the aquatic environment of central Cheshire into confusion!

I put an advert on Gumtree but it was taken off as it was an amphibian, which I thought was one of the options allowed. I rang 'Aquatics to Your Door' and asked the manager for a suggestion. Friends suggested Chester Zoo.

The bulletin board at work was my next thought. I contacted Nicola to see if she could put some details up and she said 'no problem'. I wrote out the description for her. *'Free to a good home, outgrown current tank. Warning, it will eat small fish.'* Dad wanted me to add 'hours of endless entertainment and fun'. I resisted.

I got a quick response only the next day. It was from a girl at police headquarters. 'Have you still got...' Apparently, she had had them before. Someone else texted but I offered to the first and arranged to leave it on my doorstep at seven o'clock the next evening, mindful of lockdown precautions. The next challenge was to catch it. Dad came at half six to help but we couldn't find the net.

'She's on her way,' I told Dad. 'Her boyfriend's driving her. You're going to have to get it out some way!'

'What do you expect me to do?' asked Dad.

He got the scoop from the Vanish powder for the washing machine. For one awful moment I thought he'd cut the creature's hand off!

'My frog's disabled!' I cried out.

'Give her 25% off, then,' replied Dad drily. 'Where's the tub?'

I bet no one else was doing this in lockdown. I really wish I had videoed it. Eventually, the frog was securely in the tub, all hands and feet in place. Dad passed it over through the window.

Later, I thanked Nicola for putting the ad up.

'That's ok. I didn't put the picture up because I thought that it would put people off!'

Helga and Mum cleaned the tank thoroughly, getting rid of all traces of the previous occupant. I hadn't been put off in any way. I love keeping fish and searched around for more.

'Aquatics to Your Door' were booked to deliver new species. I thought that it was a really cool idea, despite the £22 delivery charge. I had never used an online retailer before. They give you a selection of creatures. They might give you Balloon Mollies, for instance, and I won't know what colours they are until I open the package. I ordered seven fish and a couple of dwarf frogs, along with some plants. I was so excited! Mum couldn't believe I'd gone down this road again.

As there were no plants available I got an extra fish and three frogs instead of two so called them Hannah, Jessica and Naomi. I couldn't tell which was which so I decided to wait to see which died first! I have to feed them blood worms which I store in the freezer. Another task for the PA on duty! Dad got the creatures out of the packaging for me and it was great to see the tank busy again. Through Alexa I can turn the fish tank light on. One of my PAs took a video and it accidentally went into slow motion. It was so soothing. I was transfixed and played it five or six times before I went to sleep that night. The frogs were doing something similar to breaststroke. I'm going to call the video 'Lockdown' because it is as if the fish have gone into lockdown when they go slow. You would have thought that it would have lulled me to sleep but I put 'Eastenders' on which was a stupid idea at that time of night.

It didn't take long for several of the fish to float to aquatic heaven, including a red one which had looked vulnerable with no friends. The next day it was just a carcase on the bottom underneath the filter. Such a short life for the poor creature and what a waste of money! One evening I saw that a fish had had about a dozen babies. They were so tiny and cute. I sent Dad a message to say I'd had twelve babies and he replied, 'Have you had IVF?'

I bought some male guppies and when I put them in the tank they went for the other fish. Unfortunately, female guppies are in short supply in Cheshire at my usual places. Dad googled a retailer in Anderton, near the Boat Lift. We both went and found this huge place full of fish. The man was so helpful, including telling me he'd open the front hatch so that I needn't go in. I asked him loads of questions. It was an exciting adventure after not being used to visiting a shop.

We flushed a fish down the toilet once, or thought we had. One of the PAs went found it swimming around the pan! I had to apologise for the trauma caused!

CHAPTER NINETEEN
In and Around Politics

'As I was entering the Conference someone stuck a 'Bollocks to Brexit' sticker on my wheelchair.'

You might remember me giving a talk St John's Church Hall down the road from Mum and Dad's house in Hartford. It was July 2012 and I was in front of about eighty health professionals. The subject was 'Personalised Health Budgets'. I remember a range of emotions that day. Early nerves were gradually put to one side as I warmed to my task and receiving a standing ovation at the end was a moment I'll never forget.

It was an important occasion because it was the start of something that I have greatly enjoyed over the years, which is speaking in public. This has provided a range of exciting opportunities. Back in 2018, the girl who started out in that local church hall six years earlier was invited to speak at a committee meeting in the House of Lords! I had been to the Lords before but must have been around six years old at the time.

This time I went with Mum and Barbara for a meeting of the All-Party Parliamentary Group for Assistive Technology. This is a subject close to my heart and I really enjoyed myself. Mum parked the van at Crewe Railway Station and an Uber took us from Euston Station to the House of Commons. I bought a few things from the gift shop, including House of Lords mustard for Dad and a House of Lords shopping bag. Mum bought chocolate for Jess and Naomi.

There were a dozen or so of us in an upstairs meeting room. I saw familiar faces including Chris Holmes, otherwise known as Baron Holmes of Richmond. Chris became blind as a teenager and is the only swimmer to have won six Gold Medals at a single Olympic Games. That was at Barcelona. Anna

Reeves was also there. I have known Anna for some time. She is the CEO of the ACE Centre in Oldham which aids communication in education. I saw Neil Heslop, the co-founder of Leonard Cheshire, the disability charity, and its CEO at the time. Neil is also blind and the person responsible for asking me to events such as this. He's a really nice guy. We discussed the provision of assistive technology for disabled people and concluded that we were making slower progress than we hoped for. Lack of funding was a major issue. We were trying to get more into schools, for instance, particularly in the form of training for staff who work with pupils in need of assistive technology. And that was before COVID. We talked about how assistive technology has become such a big thing for the whole nation, particularly the use of Alexa.

When I see everything going on in Westminster today I think it's so weird that I've been there several times now. In March 2017 I had been invited to a meeting in the Commons where I met Speaker John Bercow. There is more about that visit in 'Hannah Moving On'. I remember seeing Seema Malhotra MP, the lady who had introduced me in the House of Commons, on 'Question Time'.

My experience within political spheres was extended with invitations to both the Labour and Conservative Conferences in the same year that I was at the House of Lords. In an email, Leonard Cheshire asked me to speak on assistive technology in work at the Labour Party Conference in Liverpool.

I did some preparation but didn't realise how big the event was. It was in Liverpool at the Arena and Convention Centre so not far to travel which was fortunate as I had to be there early in the morning. As I was entering the Conference someone stuck a 'Bollocks to Brexit' sticker on my wheelchair. Then we went through a protest against circumcision. We had to wear a visitor's badge but when Mum arrived she had to go to a different place because she had an Irish passport. She joined a massive queue as I headed to a room inside the building.

I was on a panel with Hector Minto, the Accessibility Evangelist from Microsoft and Neil Heslop. The Shadow Minister for Disability should have also been there but had to back out at the last minute. There must have been about fifty people and a tasty-looking buffet lay at the back of the room. Dad quickly tucked in. Mum missed it because she was still in the queue.

After the talk we went into the actual hall. We got some fortune cookies with Labour policies on them. We met our MP, quite by chance. Dad knows him quite well and proudly told him that I'd been speaking. I followed the journalists round like some sad groupie. I tried to get in the background for the news pieces! I drove after Laura Kuennsberg but she is one fast runner!

Jon Snow was there reporting for Channel 4 news.

'Jon! Hi!'

'Oh, hi!'

'I've been speaking today at the conference and love watching Channel Four News!'

'Lovely to meet you!'

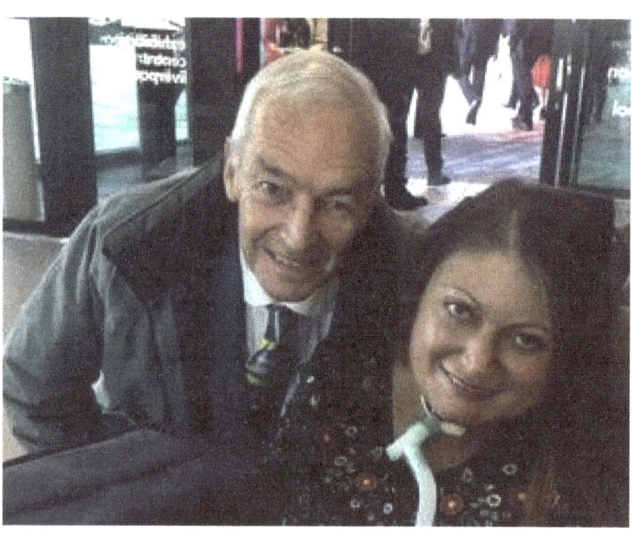

Later, we met again and he said,

'Rose, lovely to meet you again!'

I overlooked the error because he was a very nice man. We saw Boris Johnson's brother who sat next me. I don't know why he was there.

On the strength of that appearance at the Conference I was asked to write an article for a magazine. It's amazing how much has come out of events that I've spoken at. Next up was the Conservative Party Conference! This was at the swish Hyatt Regency Hotel in Birmingham. I was invited by Neil to drinks at a really posh bar. Going in I had my own drink with me but thought it quite funny that they made me drink a bit of it to prove that it wasn't bleach or anything! The seminar was put on by Leonard Cheshire and Microsoft and there would have been few longer titles in the whole conference,

'Tackling the Disability Employment Gap: How Assistive Technology Can Close The Employment Gap, Boost Productivity and Deliver The Modern Workplace.'

As well as Neil and myself there was Steve Tyler, Director of Assistive Technology at Leonard Cheshire, Hector Minto again and Sarah Newton MP, Minister of State for Disabled People, Health and Work.

It was quite an achievement to be invited to both the Conferences!

CHAPTER TWENTY
Loving the Live Music

We kept screaming, 'This is my favourite!' It was such a good night.

As you will know I love my music and there's nothing better than going to a live concert. Over the years I've seen many of the top stars and am so grateful to friends and family who have enabled me to get there and back. When I heard that the Spice Girls were touring again I just had to get tickets. It was through May and June 2019 and I desperately wanted to go with my sisters. Mum got four tickets really early on and Jess's friend Candy came with us to the Etihad Stadium in Manchester, a venue I knew all too well from watching football.

To help us get into the mood Jess had brought make-up and glitter. Mum and Dad dropped us off before going to Aunty Teresa's house to watch Tottenham and Liverpool in the Champions League. Candy met us at the ground. She wore normal clothes and told us she had smuggled some alcohol in in her pants! Jess and Naomi went over the top with my make-up but it was really funny. Candy then went to the toilet and when she returned she had the Union Jack dress on, just like Geri!

We were having loads of fun before the girls came on but the atmosphere cranked up a few notches when they appeared. We had good seats near where my season ticket was and were singing and dancing the whole time. Every time a different song started we shouted and screamed ever louder! We kept screaming, 'This is my favourite!' It was such a good night. The sound was brilliant and I couldn't fault anything.

Mum and Dad had parked down the street and round the corner. We said goodbye to Candy and Jess and met Mum who had come from the car. It was a bit of a nightmare because everyone was crowded on the pavement. As we approached our vehicle we passed a guy in his car. He shouted, 'Yow, yow!' and put out his fist for a fist pump. I couldn't believe it when Mum fist-pumped him back!

'What are you DOING?!' I asked her.

I just had to tell Dad about it when we got to the car. I love Mum when she does spontaneous things like that.

Naomi, Mum and I booked to see Ed Sheeran in May 2018. We had an extra ticket which Dad seemed keen to take. We met cousin Liz there. I've got this hilarious picture of Dad posing as a grumpy old man with a woolly hat on. He looked like he was being tortured. Huge traffic jams didn't help his spirits.

'Why did you even come?' I asked him time and again.

Concerts were worrying nights out in the first place but my friends have it off to a tee now. They always make sure that there is at least one with me at all times. Sarah and I went to see Katy Perry at the Echo Arena in Liverpool in June 2018 and that was another brilliant night. Taylor Swift was really good at the Etihad in the same month. Anna and Sarah had bought tickets for Lizzy and I for Christmas so the four of us could go and sit together. I remember having a cast on my leg after breaking my ankle. I've been missing nights like that during the pandemic.

Closer to home is the Memorial Court in Northwich which does a lot of really good productions. Jess's friend, Sophie, is in a lot of them. 'Grease' was really good. Knutsford Theatre Company often perform and they are as good as London shows.

CHAPTER TWENTY-ONE

National Heroic Service

'I'm surprised your ears weren't burning!' I told her.
'You deserve a medal.'

There has been so much coverage of the NHS during the pandemic and I must add my tribute to some of the fantastic practitioners who have kept me going over the years. There have been many appointments and countless visits to hospital and I have got to know some of the dedicated staff who have treated me as friends.

Take Dr Harris, for instance. This lady is a star! She is the dermatology consultant at Leighton Hospital but comes to Northwich Infirmary once a week. I've known her since I developed a skin condition. She is so good. She gives me the sort of attention that you wouldn't even get in a private hospital. She also likes dogs and loves seeing pictures of Mabel! Dr Harris is just amazing, getting things in motion so quickly. Having her fighting my corner makes the difficult times all the easier to deal with.

One example occurred around March 2021. I had not been feeling too good with a high temperature, mainly in the evenings. Having a temperature and not being able to cool down is just one of the hardest things to deal with for me. Things took a turn for the worse on a shopping trip in Warrington's Golden Square with Mum and Sharon, my PA. Mum wasn't sure we should have been there with lockdown looming. I remember not feeling well in the Pandora shop. Mum's friend Carolynne's daughter works there and I was swapping some charms I'd got for my birthday. I just felt like I was going to be sick and told Sharon that I needed to leave the shop quickly.

I texted Dr Harris. She suggested that I needed some intravenous therapy which I'd been trying to put off because it makes me feel sickly. The last time it had affected my enjoyment of my birthday and a visit to talk to the children at the Lancasterian School, a community special school in Manchester. I love going there. Dr Harris prescribed eight weeks of therapy. Apparently, my iron/blood level was really low. It should have been between 9 and 33. I was on 3 so she expected me to feel rubbish.

I was immediately worried about Mum having to go to Leighton regularly to pick up what I needed for my daily procedure, what with COVID being around. I knew Emma in the pharmacy in Leighton Hospital and she was always really helpful but it was still a problem in my mind. We would probably have to pick them up on Tuesdays and Fridays.

As you might remember, three years earlier, my friends Vicky and Cat had brought similar medications down when they visited me in Minehead. This was going to be my third or fourth course. You just have to make sure that they are applied within a certain time. You get a special thermometer to put in your fridge and have to add details to a folder each time a dose is given. It is a daily procedure involving a plastic bottle with a bubble in the middle which shrinks as you are having it. It takes fifty minutes to an hour. On the positive side, this was a good time to have it as I was not doing much, nor was I at work. This time a community nurse was going to be able to come out for the first occasion, to ensure that there wasn't a reaction. She was also going to be able to take care of holidays or unexpected eventualities, otherwise Mum would administer. That was really good to know. I hoped that the nurse would be Amanda who had I got to know well but had since gone to work in the community.

The process doesn't stop me doing anything but it's a hassle and makes me reluctant to eat with an upset stomach a likely reaction. It's a Catch 22 situation in that I need it but in taking it I have to be careful about the condition of my sores. However, I did feel better the last time I had a course. I hoped for the same again this time because I didn't want to be upsetting the good progress that I was making generally.

Amanda was the community nurse allocated which was a big help. She began this latest process on a Tuesday afternoon after I'd done a quick dog walk. I'd already arranged for a new PA to come for an interview mid-afternoon on that day. This added to the stress of the situation. I had about half an hour with her before Amanda turned up. I passed her on to Janet so that I could start with Amanda at about three o'clock.

I felt OK after the first dose and did singing with Choir on Zoom but during the evening I became over tired and couldn't stop crying. It was awful. I was upset and frightened. My mind was playing tricks. I had another dose at around half past ten on Wednesday morning. Amanda had to watch Mum giving it to me. I really wasn't with it when she popped in to see me in my bedroom. I went downhill throughout the day, feeling rotten. I didn't know what to do about it. I couldn't function or speak and didn't feel like myself. I couldn't even change the channel on the TV. I just sat watching BBC1 but not taking anything in. My feelings of anxiety and panic persisted. I remember the sun coming out and, typically, I would have been out in the garden straight away. I rang Mum saying I wanted to swap one chair for another but didn't have the energy. She advised against making the change, fearing that I wouldn't have the ability to guide my chair.

I needed Mum and Dad with me really badly and it felt like I was in hospital. I rang Dad on the Wednesday night. By this stage I was crying hysterically. He looked up on the internet and the nervous, stressful feelings appeared to be a rare side effect. Dad was brilliant and said that he would agree with any course of action that I wanted to take.

Thursday was even worse. I've never felt so frightened. I was prepared for an upset tummy but not feeling mentally ill. I know I can deal with quite a lot so when I can't I know it must be serious. I contacted Dr Harris and told her what was happening. She wasn't in work on the Friday but had told me that I should let her know anyway what I wanted to do.

By Friday Mum and Dad didn't know what to do. We had a chat in my bedroom. Once again, Dr Harris was brilliant. I asked if I should push through the weekend but really didn't know what to do for the best. On her day off, she still took time out to tell me to stop the course immediately. When I got off the phone I felt like crying. I emailed the haematology people. Her reaction had made us all feel a whole lot better. I really thought that she was there for me yet again but I still felt so bad about having to stop the course because it had been set up for me.

Amanda rang on the same day and was so upset for me. She had realised I wasn't myself on Wednesday but was pleased with my decision. The Haemotology department at Leighton Hospital rang me about five o'clock in the evening and were brilliantly reassuring. Everyone had been so nice.

By Monday I was feeling a lot better. Amanda came back on Tuesday to take my blood again,

'My gorgeous girl is back!!' she said. She gave me her number and offered to take swabs of sores to Leighton for me. Dr Harris rang as I was taking Mabel out. She wanted to see how I was and I told her how brilliant she had been,

'I'm surprised your ears weren't burning!' I told her. 'You deserve a medal.'

She said that I had enough to contend with every day without having all this to deal with as well. 'You definitely did the right thing coming off'.

Mentally I don't think I could have gone through the weekend on it.

I still knew that I faced an iron infusion and a reassessment of my antibiotics, maybe when my body was stronger. I just needed it sorting out. I got a phone call a few days later and an appointment was made to go to Leighton Hospital. As I travelled there with Mum and Helga I felt really pleased that it was happening. I had the infusion straight away. Helga stayed with me while Mum got me a hot chocolate and a magazine. The hot chocolate at Leighton is so good!

It didn't take long and I was home by half past five. I went on my laptop with Naomi and by half past seven I was feeling really bad again. I put my covers over me because I was freezing and didn't move until the next morning. I just didn't want to talk to anyone but Gala was really good and sympathetic. She encouraged me to drink. I knew there would probably be a reaction. I have to go again to Leighton but the next time I don't think I'll be so cheerful or excited!

A couple of days later I was still feeling grotty. The fire woman came to talk about my risk assessment for my house following a previous visit. She worked in the same building at Cheshire Police that I do. A lot of the fire people do. We had a good chat in the garden and she stayed for a while. After she had gone, I felt a bit better in the sunshine before turning chilly and needing to come inside, not feeling great. I got in my comfy chair, checked my temperature, which was really high, and settled down in front of the television. As I watched 'Hollyoaks' there was a massive bang and my television exploded! It was so loud, just like someone had been shot. The smell went through the room. It was pretty ironic just after the fire lady had left. I rang Naomi, nearly in tears because I wasn't feeling great. Dad told me to make sure the electric plugs were off. He was so good, despite being in pain ahead of his own hospital appointment. He brought a television temporarily from their house then bought another for me. It's really cool with a surrounding area light that changes. Dad couldn't wait to tell me about that!

I felt so sorry for Mum having an ill Dad to cope with as well. He was in so much pain and went to A & E. He needed kidney stones removing. I know all about stones. They are definitely one of my specialist subjects! We had a funny Houseparty while he was in Leighton, starting around half past ten after the football (City v PSG, Champions League). I knew he'd be pleased with the match and the way it had gone. Jess and Naomi joined in. Jess was in bed at the time. Stuart suddenly turned the lights out. 'Hey, I'm talking to my family!' we heard her say.

Dr Harris is a shining example of what the NHS offers but there are others who have always stepped up for me. Take

Hayley McGrory, alias the Blood Lady. I've had many blood samples taken from me over the years and, to be honest, everyone has struggled to do it. Hayley at Northwich Infirmary offered to have a go and did it straight away! From then on it has always been Hayley that I've wanted. 'Do you want Hayley?' the other nurses will automatically say when I arrive. Like other people in the NHS who I've got to know, we've become friends on Facebook. Hayley has also been to a Ronald Macdonald fundraising day at Mum and Dad's house.

Then there are the Plaster Girls. I had wanted to stand up in my chair but it wasn't properly secure. I suddenly dropped and broke my ankle. It was just before the Taylor Swift concert in June 2018. I didn't feel any pain so wasn't even aware of what I had done. I just had a bit of a headache. Next day my ankle was really swollen and we didn't immediately realise why. I had broken a number of bones. It was a bad break, the worst I've had. I was swearing like a trooper when getting my X-ray in Northwich. Mum told me to stop. The man putting the plaster on my leg said, 'Do you suffer from autonomic dysreflexia?' I asked him how he knew and he said that he used to work at the spinal unit in Southport.

For an able-bodied person they would have to pin it. They decided to put a plaster on me. I went by car to Leighton Hospital and was there for ages. I met Lisa and Lorraine, hereafter known as the Plaster Girls, and got to know them well because I was there every week for a couple of months having my plaster done. All we talked about was Love Island! I really looked forward to our meetings. It was sad when I no longer went. We are still friends on Facebook. I even took Mabel one day because they wanted to see her. She had her high viz jacket on and it took about an hour to get to the appointment because everyone wanted to stop her and fuss! I have a video of her running round the plaster room. My leg is still bent in the ankle area.

Dr Jacob at Walton knows me very well and has done for a long time, probably from around five years after I went into Alder Hey. He has done a lot of research around my issues but, sadly has moved to Dubai. He's one of many at Walton that I'm really close to. Dr Jacob has always been proud of me and what I've achieved. 'She's written two books and works at the police, you know,' he would say.

Gill with the magic fingers comes once a week for about an hour for physiotherapy. She used to be the head physio for the community physios. She has retired now but I had her name passed on and she is a godsend, as are all the brilliant medical people who I have met along the way.

CHAPTER TWENTY-TWO

Three Chairs for Hannah!

It's definitely one of the best things I've ever bought.

On Naomi's 30th birthday she had a party in Liverpool. My chair broke and I had trouble getting out of the van. Just to make the breakdown even more embarrassing it was the first time that I was meeting Dan's Mum and Dad!

I've had a bit of a chequered history with problems connected to my chairs, not least in lifts. There are examples in both my previous books! Sarah and I worked out quite recently that I had gone a whole year without being stuck in a lift-but it had been lockdown! I've had three types of chair over the years. They have been a fundamental part of my journey.

When I first came out from Alder Hey in August 2000 I just had the manual chair that I got from the hospital. I remember spending my 18th birthday inside and my friends coming round urging me to go out. We went to Rosie's in Chester. They all lifted me up the stairs! The electric one had arrived by then but I used it little for the first couple of years. I was in bed a lot and just couldn't get my head round being in it. It was so difficult to get round the idea of going out of the house in the early days. I thought it was the final straw having to rely on an electric wheelchair to get me around. 'Look at me, everyone, I am really disabled now.' Looking back, I realise how wrong I was to have that attitude because once I got used to it the electric chair gave me my independence and came into its own. It has not been without its problems, though.

I was getting into the toilet at headquarters once when the door hit the back of my electric chair and broke it. Tia managed to get me out and somehow into the lift up to my office. She was so good in a situation which showed the chair's vulnerability. I will always be grateful to her for the support she gave me at Cheshire Police. I couldn't have managed without her. When the chair broke we didn't have too many options. I rang Dad and Permobil, who are in charge of the chair, to ask what to do. It was a new model with an old headrest because I like to get used to the same one. It was affected for ages and I had to go back to my manual chair which doesn't have the same flexibility as the electric one. Using it regularly again made me think how much I relied on and liked my more sophisticated electric chair now.

The manual one has come into its own at times, however. On my Italian holiday, for instance, it allowed me to see more than I would otherwise have in an area which was hilly and difficult underfoot with lots of cobbles. It was also nice for Dad because there wasn't the stress of my electric one breaking down abroad. Also, budget airlines were not able to cope with the bigger model. When I went on holiday to Whitby I took both which gave me flexibility. It's horses for courses, I suppose.

Then there's my reclining chair. A few months after moving out of the family home I was finding it really hard to sit and relax in my electric wheelchair and needed an alternative. It's a tilting leather armchair which matches my brown sofa and it's lovely! I looked at the different colours on the internet and was delighted to see that chocolate brown was available. I was able to buy it as part of the support plan. Big items are allowed if justified. I get into it when I come back from places like Mum and Dad's and from walks. I don't know what I'd do without it. It is so comfortable and a relief from the electric chair. There is a pressure relieving cushion which you can plug into the mains.

With the reclining chair being on wheels I can get from the hoist straight into it in my bedroom. We got a manual handling expert in to explain to my team. A lot of the PAs now find it quite easy to transfer me from my electric to my reclining chair. I have my sling in already under me on the electric chair and one person can help me move which makes a world of difference. I'm not restricted. It means that Mum doesn't have to come specially.

In the summer I can use it in the garden and it is good for my sores. I can put my lap top and possum on the tray which goes all over the front and have my meals while sitting in it. It's definitely one of the best things I've ever bought and I can't believe that it took so long to sort. I remember talking to my friend Celia a long time ago about an armchair that I had at Alder Hey. She told me that I needed to get one when I moved into my new house. We didn't get one straight away but when we went to Whiston Hospital for one of my particularly difficult appointments regarding sores they advised me to get one. I really miss it when I'm on holiday. I can't get in and get snug!

CHAPTER TWENTY-THREE

The Joys and Perils of Keeping in Touch

I've rung Mo the hairdresser countless times, really wanting Mum.

The progress of technology has been a huge help over the years, allowing me to gain some degree of independence. Social media is so important for me and with technology advancing I've started to post more regularly since I've had the chance to do it myself.

I wouldn't have this house had I not gone to Birmingham in 2016 to the UK's largest disability show and become aware of the GlassOuse Assistive Device that I described in my previous book. For the first time since becoming ill I was able to use a computer by myself by fitting a black-framed device over my glasses. A combination of my head movements controlling the cursor and a bite click when it was in position gave me access to a new world, so much so that I couldn't get off it!

When Mum and Dad were away once, I used my device to navigate on Rightmove which found me this new home. Assisted technology such as this is my way into the outside world and over the years since my trip to Birmingham there have been even more exciting developments.

My Apple phone has revolutionised my life. One of the PAs put me on to the fact that anything above an iPhone 6 gives technology which allows for voice engagement. Dad bought me one. Through Siri I can now use my voice and it is so much easier. The only problem is that sometimes I'm connected to the wrong person. I remember sending a message to Mum about trousers. I'd ordered some but put the wrong ones in the package and kept the ones I wanted to send back! The message went to an old friend, Andy in Oldham. You may remember me telling you about him. Andy broke his neck whilst swimming in Goa. I first met him when I was having physiotherapy in Bury and quickly discovered that he is quite a character.

My message reached him late at night. I texted to apologise and he got back straight away. 'I'm up at six in the morning but don't worry about it. Nighty night. It's lovely to hear about you and your #trouser situation.' I still see Andy quite a lot at the football.

I can send links, photos, do emails and Facebook messages all by myself. I can purchase things on my phone with my voice. I can't believe it. It's the best thing that ever happened to me! (another best thing!!) Previously I had to put my special glasses on and get the lap top out. That was special at the time but we have moved on.

My PAs can't believe what I can do. I'm driving them mad sending them stuff all the time. Pictures, messages, GIFs. I can't stop!

WhatsApp is great fun because I can join in in every thread and conversation, on level terms. Like most people I'm in lots of WhatsApp groups. One evening in lockdown, Dad, Naomi, Jess and I were trying to find the most awful pictures of ourselves. I was on fire. It went on for about two hours. I was chuckling to myself all the time. I didn't need anyone to post a picture for me. I don't need people to write my messages any more. I have always hated people reading my messages. It's been nobody's fault but when you have your phone on your tray and a PA is near messages that pop up can easily be read.

I'm bad at using WhatsApp late at night. I'll write to Jess and Naomi, asking 'Are you up?' They will say that they are and then get quite annoyed as to why I've got in touch with them. They immediately think that at such a late hour something is bound to be wrong when, in fact, my reason for ringing is usually pretty unimportant. There was the time when I couldn't find a place on the Coast website to put my voucher (for the bridesmaid's dress for Naomi's wedding) so I rang Naomi.

'Have you just rung me for that?' Naomi said. 'You really worried me at this time of night.'

Jess got,

'Which bed should I get from Pets At Home if I was to buy a bed for Mabel?'

'You've got in touch with me now just to ask me that?'

I should in future state that it isn't an emergency if I text late.

Using WhatsApp has not been without its problems. I once mistakenly sent details of a place that I wanted to go to on holiday to the Choir group instead of my family! One came back saying how nice the place looked!

You might have sensed that I'm on Facebook a lot more now that I'm more independent. It's great to keep in touch with people from my journey such as the nurses at Alder Hey. Naomi and I share a passion for exclamation marks which I use a lot on Facebook!! I remember being told at primary school that we shouldn't overuse them. Jess keeps telling me when I don't need one. Maybe I talk in exclamation marks!!! As for Twitter, I have long spells of not doing it then I will go on randomly. I tweeted about Adele Rose, after Ant and Dec had posted their own tribute following her death.

I'm obsessed with current affairs on my apps. Siri allows me to use news apps on my phone in bed. I'll literally wake up and say, 'Hey Siri, watch BBC News on phone.' I'll be watching the news on my phone in the garden. With it propped up I can say, 'Watch BBC1 live' and up it will come. I was actually on the news when it showed the Queen's Garden Party that Mum and I attended in May 2017. I shouted to the PAs to come and look. Every time I see the Queen wearing lemon I know that my day at the palace is being featured. I spotted Mum and myself in the large crowd because I knew exactly where we were.

'You must have very good eyesight,' said Dad. I don't think that's the reason. Sue and Dave said they saw me straight away. That was the day when I told Princess Eugenie that I loved her dress and hat! When I think back I come out with so much rubbish but maybe she doesn't get too many compliments like that, probably meeting up with old people most of the time. I vividly recall chats with the Duke of Edinburgh, Andrew, Charles, Camilla... I'll stop there. It's all in the previous book!

It's good to be in the know about things and I love it when breaking news comes through. Dad and I have a competition to see who can blurt out news the quickest. Except he's got this Apple watch which is so annoying. It looks rude when someone's talking to him and he just looks at his watch. It looks like he's not interested. When I want a FaceTime with him, he will do one of three things. First of all, he will answer as an audio call on his phone which really annoys me but will talk into his watch and I can't see his face. I think he likes that because it makes him look like a spy. I will then get him on screen only for him to swing his phone round one way and the other to make me feel sick. Thirdly, he will alter the appearance of his face into an animal or some creature. One minute he is a pig, the next a dinosaur. Honestly!

Dad even works my Alexa from abroad! He has done it loads of times. He can turn my conservatory lights on and off whilst somewhere in Europe. I can just imagine him round a table with foreign colleagues saying, 'Watch this, I'm going to turn my daughter's lights off.' Sometimes I don't react, on purpose. I'm refusing to rise to it.

Being able to use Siri on my phone has allowed me to ring people independently and have more privacy but it hasn't been without its problems. I wanted to ring Danebridge Medical Centre on the way back from Cheshire Oaks. It recognised 'Dave Mitchell' who was out and it went on to his answer machine straight away. It can leave up to a five-minute message and did! I can leave a message if I need to but can't hang up so have to stay on for five minutes.

I've rung Mo the hairdresser countless times, really wanting Mum. Then I have to think of some reason as to why I've rung her. On one occasion, I panicked and said,

'Hi, Mo, just ringing about some treatments for my hair!'
She replied,
'I'll set up a consultancy with one of the ladies at the salon next week!'

One of my sisters asked why I hadn't just come clean.

'Well, I've done it about twenty times now. It's so embarrassing.'

Mo sent me an emoji and said, 'I love your calls.'

I have also had to change Dad for Daddy for the same reason. Otherwise, it rings to his work phone. It's so embarrassing saying 'Ring Daddy'. Liz BM, meanwhile, comes out as Lesbian.

I normally go to bed between half eleven and midnight. I sometimes send messages to Mum and Dad. They have lots of my food in their freezer, as I can over order. I will ask if anyone is up and, usually, no one replies. On one occasion I texted to remind them to take some mashed potato out of the freezer so I could have it the next day. It doesn't go down well.

Mum and Dad were trying to finish 'The Queen's Gambit' on Netflix. It was a series which gripped many, including them. I must have phoned them about four times! Mind you, I got a similar experience when I was watching the last episode of 'Traces'. I'd timed it deliberately so that I would be able to see it out and Mum turned up unexpectedly.

'Hello, I've just walked here!'

'Have you bought some scones?' (knowing that she had made some)

'No'

'Well, why have you come then?'

I realised later that I'd been a bit horrible towards Mum, although she got a cup of tea before going home!

One night I got home and started sending videos of Mabel to our family group, over and over. I thought it was quite funny, then we got on to stupid GIFS. It was getting to around eleven when Mum typed, 'Go to bed!'. I was kind of laughing to myself. I couldn't stop! I'm on level terms in situations like that which is empowering. I love to be able to get a picture and send it. It might be something as bizarre as my fish tank, for instance. A PA will take the photograph, then I load it on to the internet and send it out.

CHAPTER TWENTY-FOUR

Thought-Provoking TV

It was so interesting that I talked it through with Joanne after we had both watched it.

I watch a lot of television that doesn't have much impact on me and have become pretty adept at pausing, fast forwarding and whizzing through the adverts and parts that I don't want. Just occasionally, a programme about disability will come on and have a profound effect on me. I want to share some examples with you.

One such was a documentary called 'Being Frank', featuring the BBC correspondent Frank Gardner who was shot six times and seriously injured in an attack by al-Qaida gunmen in Saudi Arabia in 2004. It was so interesting that I talked it through with Joanne after we had both watched it.

Gardner explored what it was like to become suddenly disabled and particularly wanted to expose aspects of disability that we never talk about. He made the point in the programme that those closest to a disabled person bear the brunt, which is definitely the case. I feel really bad on Mum, Dad and my sisters at times. The programme also showed how small things can get in the way and be so frustrating. When he opened the lift door to go to another floor of Broadcasting House for a television appearance it was already full. Wheelchair-bound, there was no way in and nobody offered him space. Suddenly he was under pressure through no fault of his own. Welcome to my world. Things like that have been a constant frustration in my life. It made me think of times when I have been held back. Wanting to go to the toilet at work might take an hour if circumstances are against me and others are in the way. It's not their fault. It's just the way it is. Another point that Gardner made was how mental recovery is harder than the physical recovery. This also resonated with me.

Then there was a BBC2 programme called 'Silenced: The Hidden Story of Disabled Britain'. The presenter, Cerrie Burnell, uncovered the hidden story of how disabled people fought back and won their freedom having been shut out of society, denied basic human rights and treated with fear and prejudice. Cerrie was born without the lower part of her right arm so her arguments were worth listening to. What she said and showed in the documentary left me feeling grateful for how much I can do now compared to the past. Born in another age I would likely have been in an institution and referred to in the most derogatory terms.

She featured John Evans who had broken his neck doing gymnastics. In 1983 he made history when he moved out of residential care for his own home and, as such, became a pioneer for thousands of disabled people, including me. Someone else wanted to go to cinemas and night clubs but couldn't. I'm so lucky that I've got friends who will do that for me.

There was a man from Stoke Mandeville Hospital talking about how becoming disabled had been the start of a new life. Getting into sport and the self-esteem coming from it encouraged him to get back to work. Stoke Mandeville was established by Ludwig Guttmann during the Second World War. Guttmann was the founding father of organised physical activities for people with disabilities. He was a Jewish man from a persecuted race who came across and helped other 'persecuted' who the Germans saw as people that they wanted to die out completely and who many here had written off. I was thinking that if he hadn't come across where would I be today? It made me think how lucky I am being able to do so much that everyone else can do. If people like those featured on the programme had not fought the cause and campaigned (like the suffragettes) massively my life today would be so much different. Yes, I have had to write off lots of things but at one time I would have been written off totally. Would we still be in institutions today if not for people like Guttmann?

Many on the programme were talking about discrimination that they had been subjected to. Thankfully, I've not faced many unpleasant people or discrimination. There were the obscenities being directed at me from a group of women when they thought that I was blocking their view of Winsford's Christmas lights being turned on in 2002. That certainly upset me and is described in further detail in 'Hannah Same Both Ways.'

There was another incident at the Leigh Arms Dog Show. I'd previously attended this event with Bella. On the day I took Mabel I met up with Vicky, Cat and Vicki. We were having a typically good time between us. Mabel was supposed to do a trick which involved pulling a coat off my knee. As I entered the ring someone behind my friends said, 'Oh, we know who's going to be the winner here.' This was a clear reference to my wheelchair and it clearly annoyed them, as well as me. As it happened Mabel didn't do anything special despite me offering her a treat beforehand instead of after. Instead, she focused on the treat too much. We won a pack with dog stuff in and a rosette for being third in Best Bitch which the family found amusing. The programme made it clear that disability is not our problem but the world's problem. How others view us is key. It is unimaginable that through all those years I couldn't have gone to work. I felt sad for those not able to experience that joy simply because of the age they were born in.

'Becoming paralysed was one of best things to happen to me as it allowed me to be central in the disability movement,' was a quote that stuck with me because I thought that it was such a lovely thing to say.

I wanted Mum and Dad to see this programme so watched it for a second time with them. Like me, they learned a lot. Before I watched it I had a basic idea of the history of attitudes to disability but didn't think back beyond my current situation all that much. Now it has given me a perspective on how much we've moved on in such a short period of time. So much has happened, even in my lifetime.

Airlines are a good example of a feature that has become so much more geared up for disabled people. As you will appreciate from my own experiences through the books travelling by air can be stressful. Things have definitely improved over the last twenty years, not least in technology, that subject close to my heart. There are fewer barriers for us.

People aren't scared to talk about disability now, an indication that the world has become more accepting. From initially not wanting to shop in Northwich I'm asking people 'Excuse me, can you get me this/that, please...' off the shelf. (before COVID, that is!) People aren't afraid to help or chat. I forget how I look when I go round. I'm in a big chair with a tube sticking out of my neck but I've subconsciously dismissed that from my mind. I'm wanting to smile and chat with people instead. I don't think about being stared at any more but it has taken a long time for me to get there.

In an edition of '24 Hours in A and E' I was surprised to see a man who had transverse myelitis, like me. He had had it for a few years and the doctors thought that he might have had a stroke. He was in his sixties. He had played golf in the morning and was due to meet his friend in the afternoon. He developed tingles in his leg and was taken to hospital. Upper body movement remained but he couldn't go home as the house wasn't set up for him. His sons became really upset when they left him in hospital each time. One of my PAs looked at him and said how different his situation was compared to mine because he had experienced more years of a normal life before being struck down. You don't get many people featured in programmes with that condition. It made it all the more interesting.

Mum and I discussed the programme with Gala and Claire, two of the PAs. We talked about how weird it was that I had walked out of my family home and into the hospital. People often ask, 'Why didn't you go to a doctor immediately when you had the pain?' Well, you just don't dream that it would pan out like this. Mum and I went swimming to try and get through it. My friends were suggesting it might be connected with my periods. Nobody had any idea about going to the doctors. I recall when I said I would look after the girls when Mum and Dad went to the football. On the way, Jess rang them to say I was crying because of the pain in my back. So many awful things could have happened. I could just have collapsed on the floor.

Eventually, the pain got so bad that I had to go.

Mum hadn't been over-worried until I said that I had one hot and one cold leg, which was different from the man in the programme. Claire said how lucky it was that there had been a garage to convert in the house, otherwise it would have meant longer for me in hospital. The programme reminded me of how Mum and Dad had searched around for the cheapest accessible van they could find to get me home from Alder Hey once a week. How I hated going back.

I remembered being put on a ward and Sue and Dave coming that first night. They are a few hours still embedded firmly in my mind. We didn't really know where we were at back then. It seems really weird, watching me get worse and worse....I was still kind of walking but no one knew what was round the corner. The medics told me that things would get worse before they got better. I will always remember them saying that. When I talk about those times now I can't believe that I'm still here.

Now they would have given steroids and other medicines because they know what to do. Science has moved on. Back then I was going downhill but clinging on to what they said about getting worse then better. A consultant from the Southport hospital said that the first two months were key. Any recovery would be within that time span. Beyond that I would not improve.

Dr Jacob at the Walton Centre wanted to introduce me to Dr Brian Weinshenker, one of the world's leading neurologists, who informed me that it was around the year 2000, just after I went in to Alder Hey, when medics found that they could slow the process by giving steroids and plasma treatment. If my illness had happened today I could have received treatment which would have lessened the severity of the illness and offered a better outcome.

'So in my case I've missed all that by a year and it's been bad luck,' I replied.

'Yes, I'm afraid so.'

'Poo'.

It's weird looking back. My PAs have asked me when I knew that I wouldn't walk again. Mum says 'And now, over twenty years later and here you are. You're surviving a pandemic, you've survived swine flu even choking on a pizza (Book One).'

There was another occasion when I became aware of someone with transverse myelitis. Mum went to Waitrose in Northwich and while she was there she spoke to an employee who had written a book. It was about his life, living with his son who is autistic. He told Mum that his wife had had transverse myelitis and had ended up in a wheelchair before making a full recovery. They got chatting and he suddenly said, 'Are you the mum of the girl who got transverse myelitis? Oh, my goodness, when my wife got ill loads of people told me of this girl in Hartford who had transverse myelitis.' He couldn't believe that he was chatting with that girl's mother! Mum bought a copy of his book and told him about my books. He was such a lovely man, apparently.

Some days later he turned up at Mum and Dad's front door with a bunch of yellow roses for Mum and one for me. He had ordered my first book and thought it was amazing. Mum went out to the car to talk to his wife, the one who had had transverse myelitis, and she told Mum that they had met some years ago when Mum had shown their son round Greenbank School. Mum gave them a copy of my second book. Someone asked me where I'd got the flowers from and I said, 'The Waitrose man'. She thought that they were part of a delivery.

We need to teach the younger generation that disability is nothing to fear but growing up in a world where the subject is given much more respect than a hundred years ago will help. I have always enjoyed my visits to schools. They are opportunities to spread the word amongst the most impressionable of audiences. It has led to some amazing conversations, project work and countless questions from the kids. Because of COVID I've missed them so much. Just before the pandemic kicked in I did get in to Cuddington Primary School, a few miles from where I live. Naomi's friend teaches there in the upper Juniors. They were having a kind of Book Week and they had seen my two previous books.

'How do you go to the toilet?' one child asked.

I was in Naomi's friend's class and it was the first time that I'd been asked the toilet question in all the schools I'd been to.

'Well, I have a little tube which comes out of my bladder and is attached to a bag at the bottom of my trousers. When I wee it goes down the tube into my bag. Everyone is really jealous of it because if I'm on a journey and need a wee I don't need to stop the car! At night I don't have to get out of bed!'

I stayed away from the poo scenario and, fortunately, they didn't ask!

'How do you get into bed?' came the next question. I had a good answer for that,

'You know those grabber machines at the fairground? I've got one on my bedroom ceiling which comes down, opens up and lifts me on to the bed.'

The pupils thought that was so cool!

There was a lot of football stuff going on at the time. When I said that I supported Manchester City half the class went 'YESSS!' while others weren't so happy, particularly Manchester United supporters. The children always get animated when we talk football. I think it's lovely that they just want to have something in common with you. It's exciting for them.

They asked some really good questions that day. They were interested in my chair. One asked about the tube coming from my neck and I explained how it was attached to my chair and helped me breathe.

They were so honest which was really good. I'm missing that. I just have to be careful that I'm not over-honest in my answers. I don't want to frighten those young impressionable minds with any of my specific details. I've covered everything from college downwards now. I get so much out of that contact and it makes my situation so much more accessible to younger ones who can pick up the right attitudes most easily I think. They are less wary and more accepting than adults.

CHAPTER TWENTY-FIVE

'It was twenty years ago today...'

I am still alive and in my own house with much to be grateful for.

The first line of the Beatles 'Sergeant Pepper's Lonely Hearts Club Band' is an appropriate lyric to quote as 23rd August 2020 marked the twentieth anniversary of my leaving Alder Hey. I picked my GCSE results up the day after. The Mitchells came round for fish and chips that evening. We had balloons and celebrated exam results for Helen and myself. It was one of the first nights with carers and I remember sitting at the table thinking how weird it was that people were ringing our bell at ten o'clock to come and start a shift through the night in a house that had always been home.

Janet, now my friend and staff member, was head of Sixth Form when I went back to school in the September. It was the first time that I became aware of her because she didn't teach me before that. When I think back now it seems unbelievable that we had tried to get me back into school so fast, within a month of leaving hospital. The school had even made a ramp for me but it was all too soon as I don't think I even managed two days back.

Twenty years on I cannot believe or understand where the time has gone. It had been May 1999 when I first went into Alder Hey and on to intensive care for ten months. In May 2019 I was with all my friends at a beautiful wedding in Italy. Normally I don't dwell too much on all that has happened over the years since Alder Hey but the twentieth anniversary did make me think a lot about how much I have gone through, met face on and achieved. Despite periods of genuine darkness when I all but gave up I am still alive, in my own house and with much to be grateful for. I wouldn't have chosen this path for myself but I'm still on it and there's loads I have yet to achieve.

On 1st July 2001 Dad sat with me and we talked about what the future held. I know that it was that day precisely because he wrote down what I said in the form of a SWOT Analysis, a familiar format where you consider Strengths, Weaknesses, Opportunities and Threats. I still have it today and it makes for interesting reading. We didn't rely on any medical or wellbeing books. It was put together from my own raw thinking, from the heart. I want to share what we came up with and show how attitudes and material things in my life have changed. In places I've added up to date comments in bold:

Strengths

a) In spite of everything else it is good that I have not had to go back to hospital other than for medical problems in the ten months that I have been at home. I would really hate to have had to do that again after being in Alder Hey for such a long time.
b) I was worried about meeting the new carers but now I am happy with all of them.
c) I think my physiotherapy has been really good. It is consistent and one of the things which has regularly happened when they said that it would which gives me added confidence. One problem unconnected with the physiotherapists is that we had a tilt-table delivered several months ago but I have not been able to go on it much yet because the correct straps have not been delivered.
d) I'm pleased about all the things that have been supplied for me, especially the environmental controls. I am really looking forward to having a power chair.

- ***There has been so much progress in this area.***

e) Mum and Dad know a lot about my care and needs so can help out a lot. I think that this is one of the reasons why I have been able to stay at home when we have had no carer overnight in the early days.
f) I really like having Jane as my tutor for German. She is very understanding and it is one of the things that I really feel positive about.

- ***Twenty years on I'm still in touch with Jane. She'd buy me a KFC every week on the way to seeing me in hospital!***

Weaknesses

a) The relationship with the Complex Care manager.

- ***Best left there.***

b) I find it quite hard when my Mum is doing a lot of my care because it tires her out and she has a lot to cope with anyway.

- ***This has been a recurring theme through the twenty years. To this day I still worry about the strain on Mum and Dad but not nearly as much.***

c) I don't like the way the shifts are arranged around when Mum is free as it would be nice for her to have some time to herself.
d) I would like to have the computer sorted out properly. My own computer is not powerful enough and it would be good to have a new one. The man from AbilityNet came to see me and said that he would be in contact again in a couple of weeks. That was over two months ago and I haven't seen him since. It upsets me when people say they will do something then break their promises.

- *This is still a common and annoying complaint that I have. Being let down when promises are made is difficult to cope with. Life is hard enough for me without others making it unnecessarily harder. On a positive note, the computer has become a vital part of my life.*

    e) I get quite worried when people are on holiday, wondering who will cover the shifts.
    f) I want my mum to be able to relax when she's not working and caring for me as it wears her out.
    g) I feel that there are more hours of care needed but I'm not sure about having a full-time nurse here between nine and five every day. Some felt that I needed a registered nurse overlooking everything but I think it's too much.
    h) I feel that there has been a total lack of training for the carers on lifting and handling. I feel uncomfortable when I ask the carers to lift me on to the bed, as I know that this is not allowed. I don't know of any alternative.
    i) I wouldn't feel confident if Mum and Dad were away overnight. I don't like it when I'm left alone with people who aren't signed off as fully trained. This is unfair on the carers. I'm not sure how they get signed off but it doesn't seem as if they have to demonstrate a skill completely to get signed off.

- *Mum and Dad have now been across the world without me!*

    j) I feel that nobody wants to take control of me medically. When I got ill in March with my tummy there did not seem any urgency to sort it out.
    k) I know that I said I didn't want 24-hour care but would feel happier if there was someone we could call on in an emergency to help either the carer on duty or Mum and Dad (if I needed putting in bed, for example).

- *In my new home we have set-up an on-call system to support the night shift should there be an emergency. We have used this system several times since. That's not a lot, thankfully, but I was glad to have something in place as an insurance.*

Opportunities

a) In the future I would like more independence but it is difficult to think so far ahead while I'm still unhappy and uncertain about what will happen to me. I would like more say in the package and the rota. In the future it will be good to have a few people doing more hours and who I really get on with. I would like them to be part of my day-to-day life as personal assistants.

- *Significant progress. Now living independently with an established team of personal assistants!*

b) I would like to go to college sometime in the future but it is difficult to be specific about this.

- *Box ticked! Degree studied for, including time at college, and achieved.*

c) I like where we live now but it would be nice to have somewhere where I could have my own living area apart from everyone with a place where the carers could be when not needed.

- *Nailed this one! Moved into my own house in 2017, with a dedicated room for my PAs.*

d) It would be nice if simple procedures could be arranged at home without me having to travel all the way to Southport for them.

e) I know that I should be able to come off my ventilator more and do lots of other things but at the moment don't feel motivated enough to try. However, I do see that in the future it will allow me more independence.

f) In September I would like to do more GCSE's or study for another 'A' Level but I still have problems using my computer and turning pages of books. It would be good to get further help with these things.

- *Further qualifications have been studied for and passed. I did German, Law and General Studies 'A' level spread out over three years at Mid-Cheshire College. I started studying for Biology GCSE but it proved tricky with the practical side.*

g) I would like to do further computer training for things like internet surfing or writing letters. I went to the ACE Centre in Oldham last year and found it really helpful but nothing more has happened since. The speech therapist was supposed to be sorting this out but we haven't heard any more for nearly six months. I would like to try new things to help me use my computer but even though my dad has helped me a lot he is really busy and I think it would be easier to have someone teaching me on a regular basis.

- *I have done all that with help from the ACE Centre and Dad.*

h) I have seen TV programmes about dogs which can be used for helping disabled people. It would be good if I could look at that option sometime in the future.

- *Along came Bella, then Mabel! Both have enriched my life.*

Threats

a) I would like a nurse to be here to keep the carers fully trained and to look after my medical needs. However, I am worried that if she is given long hours every daytime, it will mean rearranging the carers hours and this may mean that they will get fed up and leave. I may also get fed up seeing the same person here every single day.
b) I am worried that carers are going on courses that are not wholly relevant to myself before they have been fully trained to look after me. I am worried that they will get their qualification and leave me and I will have to keep getting new carers every few months. I don't want all the carers to be 'nurses'. I want a nurse that can do that sort of thing but I want the carers to be just what they are-people who look after my day-to-day social needs.
c) I am worried that if too many carers leave I will have to go back into hospital. I really do feel that there needs to be a back-up carer to call out in case a carer is ill or on holiday. It's usually my mum or dad who has to stay up or stay in with me. Dad is sometimes away on business and I'm worried that if no one is available or Mum isn't feeling well then I'll have to go back to hospital.

- *I have been able to keep a stable team and recruit others when necessary. I have set up an on-call system to ensure a response if a PA is unable to carry out a night shift.*

d) I'm worried that the carers can't give any medication. I have a spray in case I get autonomic dysreflexia that should be taken in an emergency but nobody other than Mum, Dad or my Complex Care manager is allowed to give it. Also, the carers don't know how to interpret and act upon blood pressure readings that can indicate when I need the spray. There is the same problem with the SATS monitor when the alarm goes off in the night. Some people know what to do but others don't understand it and sometimes wake me up to ask me what they should do.

- ***My PAs have been given increased responsibilities over the years. They were particularly helpful during the pandemic when others were not available.***

When I first read that analysis again it almost seemed miraculous that so much had happened since we put it together, particularly in the 'Opportunities' section. If someone back then was going to tell me that twenty years on this is what I would be like now none of us would have believed it. It seems as if it was all written in a different age.

You still have to give credit for everything I had back then in the early days and months of my journey because it has carried me to this point. Remember that I had only been home for ten months when the analysis was put together. I read it to the PAs when Dad found it. Some hadn't been aware of all that progress because they were relatively new. I'm so pleased that Dad made me write it all those years ago. It's a document to put everything in perspective. We have been through hell and had so many awful movements but, reading it, the good far outshines the bad. It also shows how strong my family have been. I mustn't think too much about trivialities. Life is too short.

CHAPTER TWENTY-SIX

Milestones

Falling out of a go-kart in Wales...might seem an unusual choice

Over the two decades there have been significant moments in the journey. I thought that it was a good idea to ask my family to think of examples and between us we could come up with a list. Some of them may surprise you.

- Speaking and drinking water for the first time might sound strange choices but after such a traumatic experience it was nice to experience both these everyday activities which we normally take for granted. I should also add drinking alcohol again!
- My first trip to the shops was memorable. Initially I was reluctant to leave the house, occasionally panicking at the thought of meeting people. I thought that they would stare at me in my wheelchair. Now it doesn't bother me at all. It's a confidence thing.
- My short stay in Ambleside in August 2002 was my first time away and proved to be a huge breakthrough, exciting and scary at the same time! Other holidays would be longer, further and more ambitious but this little trip to the Lake District was huge so soon after leaving hospital. Sarah Norman, the person in charge of my care package back then, deserves a special mention because it was she who encouraged me to do things like pursue my studies and go for holidays. We found a cottage in the Lakes that was so nice. My carers stayed nearby within walking distance and the whole experience was a triumph. I got my German 'A' Level result on that

holiday. Sarah faxed it to the hotel and the paper was slipped under the door of our room. They put the news of my result on the menu at the restaurant we ate at in the evening. That was really special.
- Starting lessons at college in the 2003-04 academic year, after previously having them at home, made me feel apprehensive but was an important step on my road to achieving some sort of normality. I had to learn chunks of information and rely on my capacity to absorb details. I took exams at college, dictating every word for GCSE and A Level. I just don't think that I could do that now. It's so easy to forget that I've been to university, graduated and got a job.
- Tenerife in August 2005 was our first holiday abroad. I'm still getting cards from Magdalena who looked after me over there. All credit must go to Mum and Dad for finding that place. It must have been so scary for them without any carers with us, although there was a doctor and support on the site. It was the first time back on a plane with all the problems that might bring.
- Dad and I going to see Robbie Williams at Roundhay Park in Leeds in 2006. Dad was reluctant to go but Mum had an Ofsted inspection at her school. I think he was more impressed than he thought he would be!
- Falling out of a go-kart in Wales might seem an unusual choice but it convinced Dad that I could actually do some fun stuff and didn't need to be wrapped in cotton wool.

Instructor   'Use the throttle'

Me   'What's the throttle?'

That was the point when the instructor realised that I didn't know anything about cars!

- Getting a work placement with Cheshire Police in 2008 was a huge breakthrough. They opened a door for me at

headquarters and gave me a foothold. It started as a Job Centre visit but it led to so much, professionally and socially. A work psychologist did an assessment which suggested the police as a possible career. She spoke to Veronica Milligan at Cheshire Police headquarters. Veronica was their disability co-ordinator and invited me in. I was quite apprehensive because I didn't know what to expect. She contacted loads of departments within the building and one got back offering a six-week period in the research department. Veronica broke down doors for me and I'll never forget that.
- A short walk along Chester Road with the next-door neighbours' dog, Rosie, was not very far but significant in terms of my journey. From it came Bella, then Mabel.
- Transitioning from Complex Care and starting a Personal Health Budget ten years ago gave me the chance to move on with my life in a way which suited me.
- I remember Mum and Dad going away for a night and thinking how crazy that I had got that far. Later, they were to go on holiday without me and I proved that I could manage in their absence.
- The first public talk, at St John's Church Hall in Hartford, went so well that I got a standing ovation. It was 2012 and Anne-Marie invited me. Meeting Anne-Marie was huge and now she is still in my life on the training side after starting up her own company, following an initial meeting when I interviewed her for a job as I started my Personal Health Budget.
- Using the special glasses for the computer has given me such a lift and ultimately found me a home!
- The first night at my own house in May 2017, was unbelievable considering how much thought I had devoted to setting up on my own. I didn't even feel worried and now I barely remember life before I moved here.
- Going to Italy for the wedding in 2019 was one of the best experiences.

- Getting through COVID with a team who could support me without Mum and Dad being there was a huge achievement for us all.

CHAPTER TWENTY-SEVEN

Opportunities with Leonard Cheshire

...the whole experience showed me what I was capable of doing and that made me proud.

I have given a lot of thought during lockdown about returning to work. I really miss my work colleagues. They are just the best! I'm hoping it will happen one day but, also, I'm looking at developing my talents and interests elsewhere. I know that I can deliver inspiring talks and maybe becoming a motivational speaker is a way forward. With my Media degree I can offer experience within communication.

In mid-February 2021 I received an email from Claire at the Leonard Cheshire organisation. She had previously liaised with me on the transport issue which featured the televised interview with Geraint Vincent. Her email caught my attention because she was offering me some media work. As you may be aware I have had a long association with Leonard Cheshire, going back to leaving Alder Hey. The charity aims to reduce the barriers to independent living, learning and working that disabled people face around the world. As well as my experience in media I also have strong views on employment and social care. I was really pleased that Claire had got in touch, particularly at a time when I wasn't able to work at Cheshire Police. I'm happy to do almost anything and there's a lot I can offer. Initially, the areas they asked for my feedback on were not appropriate to my experience. Funding cuts and disability hate are two subjects that, thankfully, I have had little experience of.

Leonard Cheshire kept in touch. They asked if I would do an interview with them on social care. This was more comfortable ground for me and I agreed to do it by phone with Lora. I told her what social care I receive and how I can now do almost anything during the day. I can go out with my friends, go shopping, go for a walk. My PAs have helped me mould the situation and I wouldn't have been able to leave home without that. What I had before is nothing like what I have now with a support team capable of doing almost anything for me. Lora sent it to me to read up. I made a few changes, signed a consent form and sent her a photograph of myself, as requested. A copy of the text can be found in the appendix at the back.

I then had another call from Claire. She asked if I was available for media work in July, when they were launching a nationwide campaign. She wanted me to be on the panel behind the campaign which was to ensure that the government's social care reforms work for disabled people. I would have to be on the end of a phone throughout a whole week and available for a photo shoot the Thursday before. A camera crew would be heading my way! I could just imagine what that involved. Taking ages to get myself ready and looking the part then rejecting pictures because the tiniest detail was wrong! What am I like?! Claire asked if I was happy for her to pass on my number to journalists and other media people. I was delighted to be involved but hoped that there would not be any phone calls on the Friday of that week because I'd already booked to go to Chester Zoo with Dad!

Leonard Cheshire wanted to put examples of my everyday life on their social media, such as Instagram. I went around Northwich filming situations on my phone camera. I explained how good it was to have social care so that I could go and have a hot chocolate outside a café with my dog Mabel and my PA. I did some very cheesy videos in River Island saying how much I loved shopping. They were cringy!

For the shoot the photographer Frank had to feature lots of different scenarios – getting up, around the house, going into Northwich. On the day before he came I had had a preliminary chat to prepare the way. I warned Barbara, my team leader, that she was going to be involved. On the day I had a physio appointment at noon with Gill. The cameras turned up at two.

Some shots were taken in my bedroom while I was having my hair and make-up done. It looked like we were having a whale of a time. I was concerned about a bad swelling on the side of my face and didn't want it featured. I sent Leonard Cheshire a message explaining my predicament and, despite me bringing it up, they reassured me that I wasn't being a diva. 'Act natural' was what we were told. Some pictures were taken in the living room including me on my computer. In the conservatory I was pictured chatting with Mum and Barbara.

We rang ahead to Asda in Northwich because it was in a good position for access. We all got into the car, parked behind the cinema in town and went into the store. Frank called over the staff member we were dealing with and she loved Mabel, fussing over her all the time! Mabel was rolling on the floor loving the attention! In fact, she was the star that day. It was like the shoot was all about her. Frank said he'd never known a dog who liked the camera as much. Barbara and I were filmed mooching around the store, pretending to shop. We had a deadline to keep to but being with Mum she knew every other person in the shop and had to stop and chat!

Frank's shots really captured what I do when I'm out with my PAs. The staff in a café just across the way were so welcoming and we sat down there. Fran knew even more people! I was pictured getting back into the car. It had been a lot of fun but exhausting at the same time. We were involved for about three hours. Above all, the whole experience reminded me of what I was capable of doing in my everyday life and that made me proud.

Through Leonard Cheshire I nearly netted an appearance on Channel 5. I was asked to do an interview on employment opportunities for disabled people. I was all prepared. The channel rang the day before to see if I was ready, then half an hour later sent me a WhatsApp telling me that they didn't want me anymore because I wasn't in financial hardship. That's just ridiculous. How did they know the details of my bank account? Jonathan Sim, the Communications Manager from Leonard Cheshire, texted me back and joked, 'Sorry for that, Hannah, but you are obviously just too much of a success story!' That really hit home with me and reminded me of how much I had achieved.

Almost immediately, I'm getting yet another call from Leonard Cheshire, this time to be involved in a debate about employment and disability on Radio 4! It was to support their argument that the stigma being faced by disabled people trying to get work has been accentuated by the pandemic. It went out live on the 'You and Yours' programme on 11th November 2021 and I was able to talk about my positive experience joining Cheshire Police despite having a physio session with Gill at the time! Considering that and the sound of the ventilator in the background I didn't think that I came across too badly!

There was a Zoom call beforehand to talk about what would be happening but Radio 4 didn't ring me until about twelve o'clock on the day. From that point, I had to be ready to go on air and listen to the show at the same time. It was strange to be listening to the radio and hearing a voice from the studio at the same time, 'Hi Hannah, shouldn't be long now.' All the while I was having physio! I thought I came across well and seemed to get back into my media mode easily. I got across how brilliant Cheshire Police have been but hadn't really finished what I was saying about still being in work because I thought the presenter would come back to me. She didn't but not to worry.

Because of the late notice, I didn't get chance to tell many friends and family about the programme beforehand but a surprising number of people heard it anyway and let me know. I got an unexpected email soon after the programme finished,

Dear Fran,

Much water has gone under the bridge since that wonderful day at Buckingham Palace. Betty and I have often spoken about you and wondered how you were doing. It was lovely hearing Hannah speaking on 'You and Yours' this afternoon. You must be very proud. Please give our love to Hannah.
With best wishes,
Sue and Betty

They were the two ladies who sat next to us at the Garden Party when the Queen and members of the Royal Family walked past! Mum replied, sending a recent picture of us on a dog walk.

A few days later I got a WhatsApp saying, 'Morning cover girl'. It was from Jonathan Sim at Leonard Cheshire. I once told Naomi that Jon was my agent! 'You're so full of yourself, Hannah!' she replied. Anyway, Jon was drawing my attention to the i newspaper which had a picture of me and my team on the front cover! It made me look as if I had my own army and then I saw the headline, which actually included 'Britain's Hidden Army'! I just thought that was such an appropriate headline!

Inside was an article and another picture. It wasn't a complete surprise to me. The paper had wanted something positive about social care and what disabled people can have in their lives. I was really pleased with the article. The journalist who I did it with, Aasma Day, had been really nice. Jon added that Liz Kendall, the Shadow Social Care minister, had tweeted about me,

'If you want to understand real challenges in social care and the reforms Govt should actually be pursuing, please read this piece in @independent. Esp pleased to see focus on Personal Budgets which have huge potential and must be at heart of White Paper.'

Aasma did a great job and reading it made me think that things are perhaps as good for me as they can be.

CHAPTER TWENTY-EIGHT

Back to the Seaside

Even after all these years we hit a new intensity.

I started to feel poorly on the evening of Dad's 70th birthday meal in Liverpool and got worse over the following week. Mum and Dad were going away for the weekend to celebrate their Ruby Wedding. By the time they returned I was really struggling with a high temperature. I couldn't even string sentences together. We discovered a mark on my bottom. It had appeared suddenly overnight. I was crushed and my heart sank. Sores are the very bane of my life anyway but this one had been avoidable. Simply put, my cushion had been put on back to front on my chair. No one was to blame for this but it still made it all the more heartbreaking. It set me back physically and mentally.

I was so upset. I rang Mum on the Monday morning to say that the nurses were on the way. Mum told me she couldn't come down because she thought that she had caught COVID! The District Nurse found me in such a distressed state but was really nice. She told me not to worry and to stay on my bed as much as possible. At times like this I just needed my mum and not being able to see her was just the worst news. Mum confirmed that she would have to isolate for ten days.

I didn't want to continue with my life. I felt that bad. The PAs were brilliant, once again. Anna sent me a message thanking me for a birthday present and asked how I was. I told her that I didn't want to be here anymore. She replied saying, 'Do you need sympathy, a hug or wise words?' Then she FaceTimed me. I was distraught.

Over the next few hours she must have spoken to the other members of SHARKK because she organised a Zoom call involving them on the Wednesday night. I have never been as open and honest with them as I was that night. I felt so down that I couldn't put on an act any more. We were all in tears. They told me that in future they didn't just want to know about the good things in my life, they needed to know about the bad as well and perhaps I had been guilty of sugar-coating my situations in the past. It was such a refreshing conversation.

My friends were there to pull me through and the frankness of the discussion was key. Even after all these years we hit a new intensity. It wasn't just about me. They were saying that we all need to share our problems with each other. They sent me a relaxation package. That was so nice of them.

Anna rang when I was on my bed. She was at the front door with some sunflowers! Rosanne came with Benjamin for the first time. I've seen Susan and her baby Isabel. What good friends I have!

I had already arranged a second visit to Whitby and there was no way that I was not going. I'd been waiting all year for this. It was so good to have something like that to look forward to after a troubling time. I was excited but nervous as I'd not done anything for a month. My body was quite weak because I'd been on my bed so much but I was determined to go. Jess and Dad arranged to meet us there. Sharon, my PA, took her collie Tess for the week while Naomi and Dan were bringing Betty, the day after. She's really grown now and is as laid back as her parents! I love her scruffy coat. She's turned out to be the perfect dog for them and was a real bonus of the week. Claire came for the week from my team.

We stayed at the same places as last time and started with a takeaway which somehow got lost amongst the surrounding farms. The next day we shopped and mooched around Whitby. Mum stayed behind and Betty chewed the door stop and the first page of the property's information booklet!

On Monday I fancied going down the coast to Bridlington but got stuck in loads of traffic. Time there was limited. We walked on the pier. I bought a snow globe, naturally! We had to get back for a booking in the famous Magpie Café on the harbour. We left the dogs behind but they were fine. I remembered from before that I had to go through the takeaway part of the property into a lift to access the café. The lift door didn't shut properly when Dad and I got in. The lift wouldn't move. What is it with me and lifts?! Dad picked the intercom phone up. 'Hello... hello.' It was a surprise when Naomi answered it, 'Where are you?'

'What are you doing answering the phone? Do you work at the Magpie? Is there something you aren't telling me?' I said.

Dad slammed the lift door shut and we got to the table. We ate such a nice meal with huge amounts of fish. Mum had given the waitress a birthday cake for Dan and she came out to announce his birthday. Daniel is so shy but seemed to quite enjoy the restaurant singing to him!

I noticed newspaper in Mum's fish portion and remembered the last visit when I'd seen that my birthdate was on my piece underneath my scampi. I thought it had been a sign back then. Not so. It turned out that all the papers had the same date because that was when the restaurant opened in 1939! The fish shop takeaway was shut and locked when we went back down in the lift. Naomi shone a torch through the window to see where we were and someone came to ease my embarrassment!

Peasholm Park had been a highlight last time so we headed back to Scarborough the following day. It started raining but we enjoyed our visit. Dad loves Peasholm Park and wants to come back when the war games are operating!

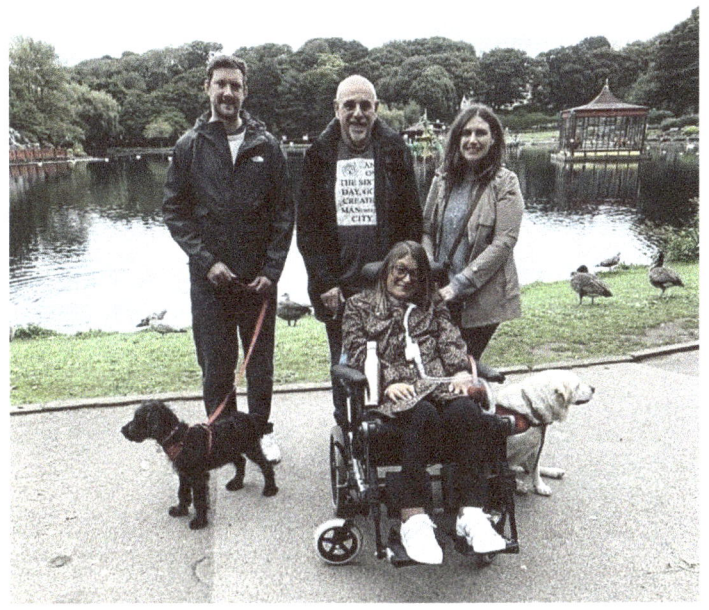

On Wednesday we met Mum's college friend, Joan, in Pickering at a Garden Centre. I spent most of the time with my back to them (not on purpose), talking to a lovely couple called Bob and Joan who were staying in Staithes. They were asking a lot about my disability. Their son had been murdered and they talked about how every day is important. I talked about Italy and other quality experiences that I'd had.

Then it was on to Sandsend, a small fishing village just north of Whitby. I had never been before but it is now my new favourite place! I really wanted to take Mabel on to the beach and determined to the next day. We had a look at gift shops and enjoyed an ice cream in the sunshine. We ate at our house in the evening, cancelling a proposed meal out. Mum and Dad were able to watch City win 6-3 in the Champions League. The next day the tide was in at Sandsend so Mabel was denied her run! We went to a café and had a lovely snack in the sun.

The PAs joined us for a gorgeous meal in old Whitby the next day after I had been to a jeweller's shop that I wanted to visit. We were out for nine o'clock on the last morning which never ever happens! We had a brilliant time and were able to tell the owners personally as they turned up before we left! We headed back to Sandsend where Mabel finally got on to the beach!

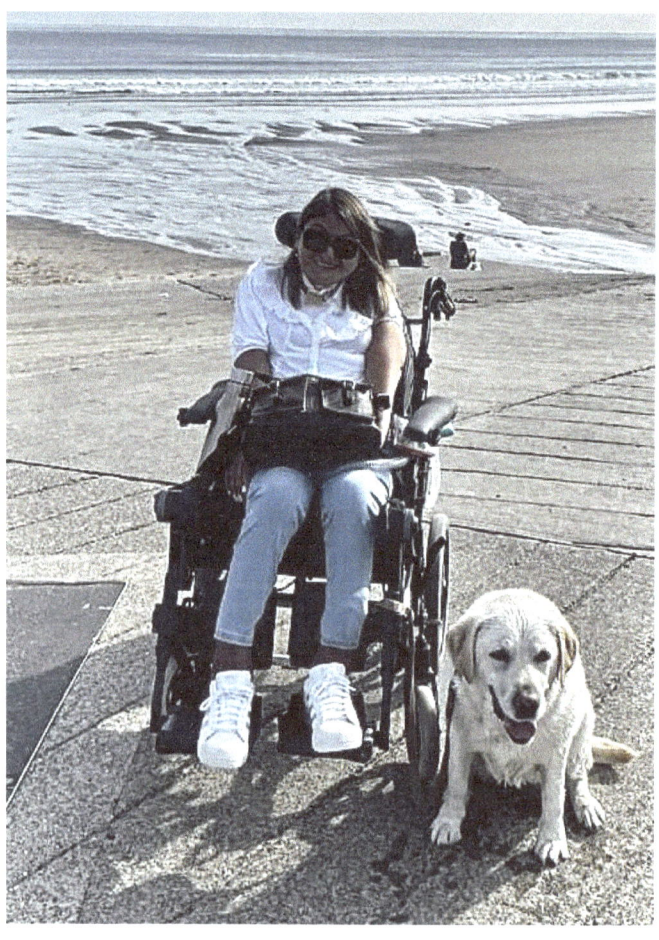

CHAPTER TWENTY-NINE

Meeting up - at last!

Joanne came with her mum and the meeting was lovely.

A holiday in Whitby and the recent media opportunities with Leonard Cheshire are examples of events that I would not have even considered doing twenty years ago. Despite my obvious setbacks and fluctuating fortunes health-wise I continue to be grateful for all the special, often unexpected experiences that have been part of my life as a disabled person. I savour the quality that they bring and I store each in the happy memory bank for those times when I'm feeling down. I have met royalty, spoken in Parliament, holidayed abroad and moved into my own house. I have been supported by wonderful friends and just the best family ever. Before I finish I'd like to share three recent reasons to be cheerful.

A trip to Tatton Food Festival might not seem that special because I have attended shows and festivals like it many times over the years. This one, however, was different because it showed me that, given the right circumstances, I can experience and almost touch normality. It was 2021 and significant for the fact that I was with Naomi, Dan, Jess and Stuart for the first time as a five without any PAs or parents.

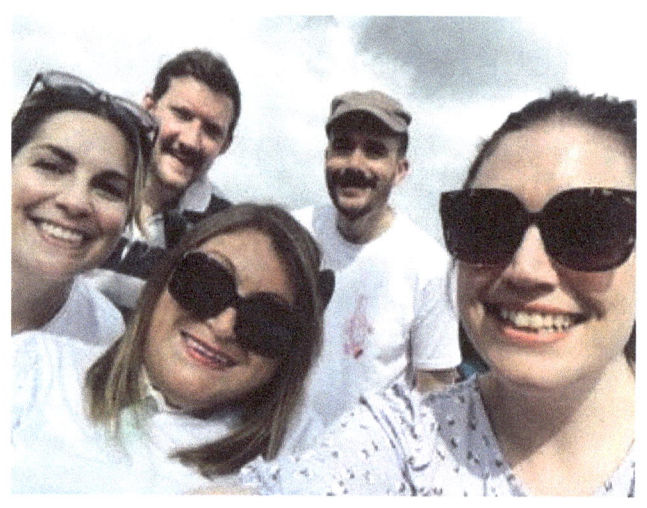

I think Mum and Dad were a little apprehensive because of the size of the Tatton Park site, just outside Knutsford. I was most concerned about the chair and how easily I would get round.

It was a test but we had a brilliant day. Naomi drove and Jess and Stuart met us there. We got really close to the action for half price and the ground was, thankfully, firm enough. A good start. The current Masterchef winner, Tom Rhodes, was demonstrating. I had a good view and was happy being left on my own. When the demonstration had finished, I got into 'picture with celebrity' mode. Jess was back by then and reluctant to take it, having seen this happen so often. As everyone was coming out of the demonstration, I drove my wheelchair up to Tom. He told me that it was his first public demonstration since becoming the Masterchef winner. One of the other finalists then came out and I asked for a picture with her, much to Jess's greater annoyance. 'Are you happy now?' she asked me after I had posed.

We bought food, drink and loads of goodies and had so much fun. It was really relaxing and we didn't have to worry about the time. We listened to some of Sophie Ellis Bextor's set but didn't want to hang around at the end as a lot of people would be leaving at the same time.

Naomi and Jess had the duty of emptying my leg bag. Naomi wasn't keen so Jess took it on and got it down to a fine art. The bag was full when we got back into the car. Jess told Naomi to empty it as she was nearest. She hadn't used this type before and there was wee everywhere, over their hands, over the car! Despite that, I can't believe what a nice day it was. It was something like a normal day and that is as big an accolade as I can give it.

As you will have worked out Joanne has been such a big part of this chapter of my life and we have been looking forward to meeting up for so long. It would be far from simple with the mileage between Cheshire and London and the many issues that we both have to overcome. However, a plan emerged and we agreed to meet half way at the BBC Good Food Show at the NEC Birmingham. Thursday, 25th November had been written large in my calendar of events for weeks as the day finally dawned.

Circumstances tried to conspire against me up to the last minute. We had removed a dressing on my back and I was a bit concerned but we had planned to go to the show that day and I didn't want to miss the opportunity. Everyone was saying to me, 'Hannah, get in the car and go to the show.' They realised how important meeting Joanne was to me.

I took that advice and went with Mum and Dad. We got there first so went in and had a look around. We heard that Joanne had managed to get near us in the car park which was amazing at such a big place. I had texted her beforehand to say that it cost £16 to park.

Then I got a text to say that they were outside and I was so excited! I asked Mum and Dad to get the video ready to record the meeting. Mum did it. It's quite funny but I kept telling her she was doing it wrong. Haphazard would be a good way of describing it.

Joanne came with her mum and the meeting was lovely. Her mum sounded just like she did on the phone, which isn't surprising I suppose! Joanne couldn't see me so I described what I was wearing. I couldn't believe we had made it and neither could she. We had been talking about doing it the previous year but couldn't because of COVID. 'Maybe we can do it next year,' we had said back then. Joanne had broken her ankle, we didn't know if her mum would be free, I had my sore. So many factors were at work but they didn't stop it happening!

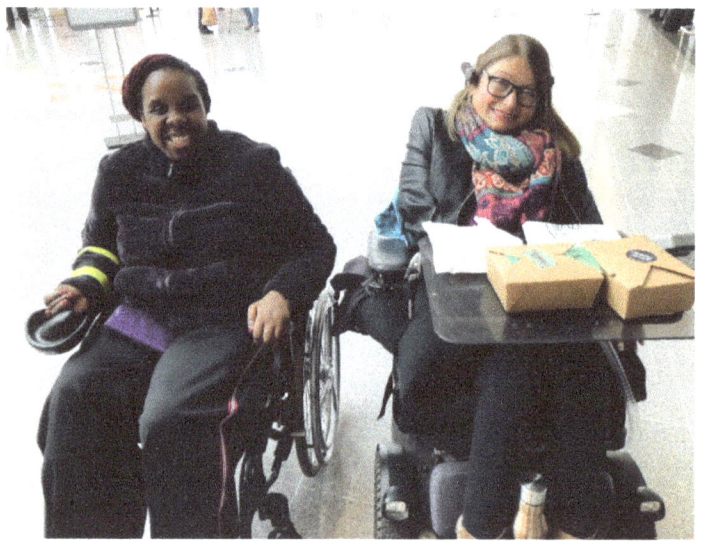

With my lovely friend Joanne

We sat and got a drink at a table with our parents. Dad bought brownies, then the parents went for drinks and the two of us were able to talk together. We agreed that we needed more time next time. We were together for a while around the show but there were too many distractions. We probably had an hour together in all. It was so good! We have talked further on the phone since then, still disbelieving that we had met.

I bought too much stuff at the show but there were some lovely purchases. Looking round the stalls I heard a voice saying, 'Hi, Han'. I thought to myself, 'Oh my goodness, who can this be?' It was the woman who does the pebble art in the

Northwich Artisan Market. 'That's so weird,' she was saying, 'You turn up everywhere, don't you!' 'Yes, I do.' It was a costly meeting because I ordered a new picture which I will be able to pick up in Northwich.

Joanne and I have often talked about how good it would be to have a holiday home to go to regularly. Originally, I wanted this to be abroad in the hot sun but have limited my ambitions through COVID. Spending a lot of time on my bed recently I was able to take my mind off things by looking for properties that might suit my needs. Well, after much research it has finally happened! Mum, Dad and I visited a number of sites in England and Wales and have chosen a lodge in beautiful Snowdonia which will be set up for my specific needs. It's got three bedrooms and overlooks Zip World. I can't wait to spend time there with my family and I'm sure you'll be hearing lots more about it!

CONCLUSION

It's the simple things that I often miss the most. I was in my kitchen one day and said to Dad, 'I wish I could write something down.' I wish I could stroke Mabel and give my family and friends a hug. I try to remember what it felt like to do such things that others see as normal.

I have to make the most of every day. None of us knows what's around the corner, including me. Life hasn't dealt me a good hand in some ways but there will be many people who haven't had such a rich variety as I have. As someone once put in a letter to me,

'Hannah, you have achieved more in your twenty years since you came out of hospital than many will in a lifetime.'

Over this period I've come to realise that this is me. I cannot change the situation. I am the person that I am now because of everything that has happened. I don't have to mask what I feel any more, emotionally and physically. What you see is what you get! I am Hannah unmasked.

APPENDIX

Interview with the Leonard Cheshire organisation, 2021

What social care support do you currently receive?

I employ care workers for my health needs to enable me to get on with my day-to-day life. They drive me to work and support me with meeting up with my group of friends and with shopping.

My social care is really my arms and legs! It enables me to live a fulfilling life, so I don't feel restricted. It enables me to socialise. I am very lucky as I get to do lots of things just like anyone else.

I have a dog called Mabel, she's part of the package, so effectively she has twelve owners! My care workers help me with housework, gardening, cooking meals – in fact they help me with everything.

They even come on holiday with me which is amazing! I have been to Florida and travelled to Italy for a best friend's wedding, which I wouldn't have thought possible. It is lovely for me to have my own support to enjoy my holidays.

How often do you receive it?

I have 24-hours a day support. I have two care workers in the morning who support me to get ready for the day. I have one care worker throughout the day and the same in the evening.

Do you receive all the support you need?

I do but it has taken a long time to get it exactly how I need it.

Has your care package been affected by the pandemic?

During the pandemic I didn't get enough advice on how to deal with PPE for my care workers. I felt left to my own devices which was a bit scary as I was responsible for a large group of people. The amount of care I received wasn't compromised.

How does social care support impact your life? What benefits does it bring?

Social care gives me the freedom to live the life I want to live, to do what any other able-bodied person can, or wants to. Without social care it just wouldn't be possible. I would be reliant on my parents. Social care gives me more options to see my friends, go to work and be independent. I moved out of our family home four years ago which was a big step, but I now feel I have true independence.

I feel incredible! I feel very lucky and independent, and things are the best they could be in this situation. Having a disability makes you feel restricted in so many ways, but, if you have good social care, it changes your life forever. It has taken years and years but now I have all the good social care I need.

Can you think of an example where social care has made a difference to your life?

One of the biggest differences social care has made to me is independence. I can now live independently and socialise with friends and I have a job. It is that sense of flexibility and control that is important.

Social care enables you to have flexibility and independence from parents and that's really important for me. I just want to live the life I would have lived regardless of disability. I have achieved big goals. I work two days each week at police headquarters. My care worker stays at work, so if I need anything they are there and ready to enable me. I have my own transport which helps me get out and about and go to work.

What would your life be like if you didn't receive your current social care support?

I'd hate to think! My parents would be doing a lot more than they are now! The fact that I can do with my days whatever I choose is amazing and Mum and Dad have their own lives. I haven't had to rely on them. Life would be very hard without social care; it wouldn't be very enjoyable without my independence.

What does good quality social care look like to you?

It is about having someone that can be with you, enjoy things with you and enable you to live the fullest life you possibly can. You don't have a lot of choice in other aspects of your life. The choices social care brings are imperative.

What changes would you make to the social care system to improve it? And why?

More credit should be given to care workers, they don't get the credit they deserve! It's the most important job in the world to me and my family. My life wouldn't be the same if it wasn't for them. I want to shout from the rooftops that care workers need more support and recognition.

Social care needs to be more accessible. There are a lot of people that don't have access to the support they need. It needs to be readily available for everyone.

What aspects are most important to get right? (e.g. affordability, quality, ease of setting up, equality of access, flexibility etc)

Ease of setting it up, you need a good support network around you and you need to be able to talk to someone who has that experience. You need to find the right people to enable you to access social care.

How do you think improvements to social care can be achieved?

By talking to the people that need it and listening to what is important to them. Social care needs to be looked at individually and tailored to individual needs.

How would you describe social care to someone who doesn't know or understand what it is?

Social care is about supporting needs but not just focusing on health. It should support every aspect of life including socialising and going to work. It is an all-round type of support. It should be a holistic approach to enabling someone to be independent and give them back control of their life. The individual must be at the heart of situation.

Is there anything else you would like to tell me about your thoughts on social care?

My life has changed dramatically for the better because of the social care I use. It's enabled me beyond my expectations. I feel very strongly that others should have that control and independence if they choose.

Lightning Source UK Ltd.
Milton Keynes UK
UKHW022307160522
403082UK00006B/440